The Love~Powered Diet

The Love~Powered Diet

WHEN WILL POWER IS NOT ENOUGH

Victoria Moran

NEW WORLD LIBRARY
SAN RAFAEL · CALIFORNIA

All suggestions in the book, dietary and otherwise, are intended for healthy adults. The author is not directly or indirectly dispensing medical advice, or prescribing the use of diet as a form of treatment for disease without medical approval. It is not the intent of the author to diagnose or prescribe. The intent is solely to offer information. You are encouraged to work with your chosen health care provider on any dietary or lifestyle changes you undertake. In the event you use the information herein without the approval of your health practitioner, you are prescribing for yourself, which is your constitutional right, but the publisher and author assume no responsibility.

The Twelve Steps and brief excerpts are reprinted with permission of Alcoholics Anonymous World Services, Inc. Permission to reprint this material does not mean that AA has reviewed or approved the contents of this publication, nor that AA agrees with the views expressed herein. AA is a program of recovery from alcoholism—use of these excerpts in connection with programs and activities which are patterned after AA, but which address other problems, does not imply otherwise.

LIBRARY OF CONGRESS CATALOGING-IN-PUBLICATION DATA

Moran, Victoria, 1950–
    The love-powered diet : when willpower is not enough /
by Victoria Moran.
      p. cm.
    Includes index.
    ISBN 0-931432-75-8 (acid-free paper)
    1. Compulsive eating.   2. Reducing diets.   3. Obesity—
Psychological aspects.   I. Title.
RC552.C65M67   1992
613.2'5—dc20   91—30718
                                                  CIP

Permissions will be found following the index.

Published by New World Library, 58 Paul Drive, San Rafael, CA 94903

ISBN: 0-931432-75-8
First Printing, January 1992
Printed in the U.S.A. on acid-free paper

10 9 8 7 6 5 4 3 2 1

To

My Daughter Rachael

Who Shows Me Every Day

What It Is

To Live in the Present

And Love Without Question

Table of Contents

Acknowledgments

All books are probably collaborations. A great many people certainly helped with this one. I owe its inception to a conversation I had with Marilyn Diamond while working on another project that was not coming together. I told her that my heart wasn't in it. She answered, "Things are too critical now for any of us to work on something that doesn't have our hearts. What *is* your heart in?" I started to describe this book. My heart had evidently been working on it all along.

As soon as I had put together an outline, I presented it to my literary agent, Patti Breitman. She was enthusiastic about *The Love-Powered*

Diet from the beginning and she has worked closely, patiently, and supportively with me throughout the writing process. Patti read or listened to every word of this book and offered hundreds of useful suggestions. It is a real privilege to have Patti as my agent and friend.

Patti's work resulted in getting the book proposal into the hands of Leslie Keenan, a senior editor at New World Library. Leslie and all the people at New World Library have been wonderful to me. They've appreciated the message of this book all along, and Leslie and her colleagues have done everything possible during its production to make this book precisely what my heart and I were hoping for.

While I was involved in the consuming process of turning ideas and outlines into a finished product, my dear friend Robert Morris provided invaluable help. From practicalities like the use of his photocopier and fax machine to his own practicality that helped me keep the concepts I was writing about down to earth, Bob gave of himself and his resources for over a year helping me to bring this book into being.

I am grateful to Marilyn Diamond for taking time from her busy schedule to write the Foreword for *The Love-Powered Diet*. Because her work has meant so much to me, her words are particularly meaningful. In addition, the creative people who provided the recipes from their cookbooks in Appendix B have made a most appreciated contribution.

I also wish to thank George Eisman, R.D.; Suzanne Havala, R.D.; and Michael Klaper, M.D., who read Chapter Seven, which deals with nutrition, and provided helpful clarifications. Others who gave me suggestions, synonyms, books, moral support, networking connections, clerical assistance, and antidotes to writer's block include Deborah Allen and George Eastman, Nathaniel Altman, Charles and Linda Baker, Ellen Bring, Syndee Brinkman, Christopher and Gloria Deatherage, Jay Dinshah, Ann Cottrell Free, Evelyn Gorten, Ann Hardy, Suzanne Hatlestad, David Hoch, Michael Hummell, Patrice Klausing, O.S.F., Mignon Lawless, Cheri Lin, Tina Repp, Becky Robinson, Dorsey Roe, Dolores Sehorn, Maureen Shebesta, Edythe Siegel, Elizabeth Simons, LouAnn Stahl, Suzanne Tague and Jim Jarzembowski, Vicki Unshuld, Rick Vandever, and Barbara Weiman.

Some of these people also helped me hold down two jobs—mother and writer—as this book was taking shape. Other friends who were genuine blessings in this regard include Sandra DeSai, Helene Lin, Janice Pierce, Lisa Prizio, Kim Endahl-Tsoconos, and Barbara Tuchschmidt.

Research help came from Kim Bartlett and Patrice Grenville of *The Animals' Agenda* magazine, and from Paul Obis, Jr., Mariclare Barrett Obis, Carol Wylie, Sally Cullen, and Drew DeSilver at *Vegetarian Times* magazine. Both magazines also graciously allowed me extended deadlines and a sabbatical from article writing while I worked on this book.

Sincere thanks, too, go to those who anonymously filled out questionnaires concerning their recovery from food addiction, as well as to Alcoholics Anonymous and Overeaters Anonymous for permission to use references to their organizations and to the Twelve Step program. I also want to thank everyone who agreed to be interviewed and quoted for the pages that follow, as well as those whose books and articles are quoted and the many reference librarians who helped me to locate that material.

Each individual who provided information and inspiration for this book is part of it and is special to me. Some of these are personal friends, others are acquaintances. Still others I know through my work as a writer, and some I know only through their work. I consider all of them my tutors in Love-powered living. To those who are my friends, and also to my family, thank you for your patience while so much of my attention has gone to this book. Most of all, I thank my Higher Power for giving me something to say and for showing me that Love can make quite a difference.

Foreword

This book can change your life. The methods described herein for both inner and outer change will redefine the way you think about, prepare, and eat food. It will also give you access to a serenity, peace, and joy that you may never have known before. *The Love-Powered Diet* describes a very simple, but completely radical, new way of living.

There is no need for me to add to the ideals and solutions that Victoria Moran offers to you in this book. They are impeccable, and she has done her usual inimitable job of presenting a higher level of conscious living for you to consider and put into practice. I heartfully and mindfully urge you to do so. Her recommendations work: You *can* change your attitudes so you will *want* to change your food choices.

What I *can* do is introduce you to my friend, Victoria, and add my own personal experience of this special person. Over the past few years, she has become much more to me than a friend. In my life, I count her as one of my most invaluable influences. Through *The Love-Powered Diet*, she can be that for you, too.

Victoria has so much to give, but is one of those rare people who sees that there is also something to learn from everyone. We have been able to communicate like close sisters, and have been there for each other at moments of pressure or uncertainty. She is here now to do that for you in this book.

What do I know about Victoria? Hers has not always been an easy path, yet I have never known a time when she has not been perfectly ready to roll up her sleeves and learn something new to make her life work. She has met challenges without giving in, yet she remains gentle. That gentleness is central to the message on the pages that follow.

Do you want to meet unconditional love? It's here. Do you want to know how to live it, for yourself and for others? Listen to what is advised here and let it be your guide. Your progress will *never* be judged and your effort will always be praised. Expect to lose your feelings of self-doubt and your self-inflicted suffering along with unnecessary pounds. Expect to gain a knowingness bordering on the highest wisdom, a compassion for yourself and for all beings, and a LOVE OF LIFE that is nothing short of divine.

Marilyn Diamond
Sarasota, Florida

Author's Note

The premise of *The Love-Powered Diet* is simple. It is one idea that has two parts:

1. Inner awareness of unconditional Love can make profound changes in a person's life.
2. Inner change includes the ability to make positive, loving food choices.

This book is especially addressed to food addicts—that is, any person of any body size who is engaged in a longstanding battle with a knife and fork. Its principles can, however, help *anyone* eat more healthfully and live more happily.

The format of the Twelve Steps, originally developed by Alcoholics Anonymous, is used in *The Love-Powered Diet*. These steps are not the only way to bring about a spiritual awakening powerful enough to change one's life and behavior, but they have had unparalleled success in helping people with a wide range of dependencies including alcohol, drugs, unhealthy relationships, and compulsive eating. There is no official or unofficial connection between this book and any Twelve Step organization. The way of eating introduced in this book is not endorsed by any Twelve Step organization. (Neither, for that matter, is any other specific way of eating.)

The loving food choices referred to involve selecting natural foods that promote physical health and discourage overeating. Choosing these foods expresses love not only to oneself but also to the world in general, including nonhuman animals and the environment.

The spiritual and physical aspects of the Love-powered diet are two sides of a single whole. There are many people who have overcome eating disorders by approaching food differently than I suggest. Others have made significant changes by using the style of eating discussed in the later chapters of this book without consciously taking any inner or spiritual steps.

Nevertheless, linking the two creates a winning combination. In fact, one can lead to the other. A person who deepens his or her spiritual life often evolves toward a gentler, more natural diet. Conversely, people who improve their diets, particularly those who become vegetarian, are often led to explore their spiritual natures.

Recognizing that spirituality is an emotionally charged subject for many people, I have done my best to keep my vocabulary and references nonthreatening both to people who are religious and to those not. If in any instance I have failed at this, please do a quick translation and substitute a word, phrase, or concept that is comfortable for you. You do not have to change your beliefs about religion or an afterlife to draw upon the Love already within you to make *this life* one you can live in freedom and joy.

Introduction

This is your fairy godmother speaking. You can have a body that you think is gorgeous, not just for the ball, forever. You can go to sleep at night without hating yourself for what you ate during the day, and you'll never again need to count calories or carbohydrates, grams of fat or ounces of food. You only need to count yourself lucky for having discovered the Love-powered diet.

Okay, so I'm not your fairy godmother. I'm another person just like you with a food problem that took me around the block so many times I could have passed as a meter reader. I cannot zap you with a magic wand. You'll just think I did once you discover within yourself a source of power to change your eating and your life that's more effective than a regiment of fairy godmothers marching in formation: This is the power of Love. Don't be put off by an overused word. It is an extremely under-used resource.

You know how being in love transforms the way people look and feel, and how loving someone—even a goldfish or a parakeet—can give a person a sense of worth and purpose. There's more than one story about a small woman lifting an automobile off her child trapped beneath. There is also abundant evidence of the crucial role played by love in healing. Physicians such as Bernie Siegel, Arnold Fox, and C. Norman Shealy have documented in numerous books how loving oneself and others and being willing to receive love in return can mean the difference between getting well and giving up. When patients open themselves to Love as an active energy in its own right, they can experience changes in their bodies and emotions that appear miraculous. You may think of this as divine Love, or as the synchronizing force that keeps electrons whirling about the nucleus of every atom.

However you perceive it, this Love can revolutionize your relationship with food. This is because the Love already inside you is not only strengthening and healing, it is *filling*. If you have a history of overeating and overweight—or its flipside of chronic dieting, bulimia, or compulsive exercising—you may already have realized that you're not eating to fill your stomach. You're eating to fill a gash in your soul as devastating to your well-being as the one in the ozone could be to this planet. It's what Pascal called the "God-shaped hole in every man that only God can fill." If you're uncomfortable with this reference to God, substitute the word "Love" and keep on reading.

There is not enough food on earth to fill that inner void, and there are not enough friends, lovers, or children; houses, cars, or stock certificates; clothes, compliments, or accomplishments to fill it either. Nevertheless, when you connect with Love, a comfortable sense of "enoughness" begins to emerge. Popular dictionaries do not recognize enoughness as a word, but without it, you and food will always be at war. You win this battle when you refuse to fight. Attach your willpower to the nearest white flag and let Love take over. That's when you will understand that *you* are enough. You are attractive enough!

You are lovable enough! And for this day, the only one you've got, you are thin enough, too.

Do you know what will happen when you comprehend—not just with your head but with your heart and your spirit—that you are indeed thin enough for the day at hand, that you are truly attractive and lovable? You will treat yourself as someone who is all those things. For starters, you'll eat like a thin, attractive, lovable person does. When I was fighting food with the vigor of a fresh Marine recruit, a wise old fellow told me that I was putting the cart before the horse in trying to eat less than I wanted and exercise more. He said that it works the other way around, that people who are healthy automatically do healthy things.

Goodness knows, I was an authority on healthy things. I had been writing articles about health, fitness, and beauty since I was nineteen. I read, researched, and wrote, keeping abreast of the latest trends in diet, nutrition, exercise, and behavior modification. I interviewed experts and passed their findings along. I had accumulated so much information that my head ached, but I was trapped in a binge/diet cycle so insidious that most of the time, my heart ached, too. It was embarrassing enough to go from fat to thin and back again like a human accordion. In addition to seeing myself as a dietary failure, though, I saw myself as a phony. The words I wrote were true based on the knowledge available at the time, but I wasn't able to put them into practice. Like a marriage counselor going through his fifth divorce, my work and my life were sorely fragmented.

Fragmentation—fragmented lives in a fragmented society—is a component most of the time when eating is out of balance. The Love-powered diet meets fragmentation with integration, because pure, essential Love is an integrating force. It doesn't foster bits and pieces. Love will not only make a difference in what you eat or the amount of exercise you get. It does not only have to do with how you feel about your body or how much it weighs. The integrating power of Love can bring all your parts into a functioning whole. When it infuses the way you eat and the way you live, your body will definitely show results, but so will every other aspect of your life. Nothing less than that can bring about changes that last.

When Love fills your emptiness and integrates your fragmented factions, you'll no longer need a closet filled with clothes that range from the petite boutique to the stout shop. You won't need to be a person who starts every Monday with a dismal diet that's tossed aside by Tuesday noon. You can stop spending your money on every pill, potion, and promise that comes around: the kind of Love I'm talking about keeps its promises a day at a time, just as surely as the sun brings daylight every morning. Without that, weight loss is destined to be temporary. You know that's as true as an oath in court because you've lost weight before. You'd be better off keeping the body you have right now and learning to cherish it than to have one more raving success with a diet, then blow the lid off it and despise yourself. Those episodes erode the spirit. You deserve the chance to leave them behind for good.

The only way I know to bring destructive eating to a screeching halt and keep it there on a daily basis is to let Love handle it. I not only tried the other ways, I wrote articles about them. There were plenty of good ideas in those approaches. Many were sane and logical, devised by intelligent, compassionate people, but the power to make them work for me wasn't there. They presented valid facts about nutrition or exercise or "thinking thin," but they were as useless to me as a perfectly decent battery in a flashlight that needs two.

The Love-powered diet is different because it works on both perspective and practice. On an inner level, it means trading willpower for Love's power. In practical application, it means living and eating in a Love-inspired fashion. The foods you'll prefer will be those that express love—to your physical self, to all livingkind, and to the planet that provides our food in the first place. You won't be dieting. It's been recognized at long last that regimentation cannot realistically be imposed on natural processes, and responding to hunger is as natural as blinking or breathing. Instead of dieting, you will be choosing to care for yourself and those around you as you make your selections at the supermarket and from the restaurant menu.

Because you're worth the best, your way of eating will reflect the lowfat, high fiber-and-carbohydrate recommendations of the surgeon general's report, the American Heart Association, the American Cancer Society, and virtually every legitimate study on human nutrition of the past twenty years. In fact, it will epitomize these recommendations. And luscious fruits, colorful vegetables, hearty whole grains, and legumes satisfy hunger while they discourage cravings. **With a**

Love-powered attitude and these foods as the staples in your kitchen, you can eat all you want because what you want will be just what you need. Weight loss and maintenance will proceed spontaneously without undue attention. You can stop *watching* your weight and start *seeing* the beauty that is in you and around you. Furthermore, a Love-powered diet will not only benefit you, its reduced reliance on animal foods spares natural resources and is easy on the earth. In this way, Love works *in* you to make your life better and *through* you to make your world better.

There's an old maxim that says, "He who lives for himself alone lives for the meanest mortal known." Those who eat for themselves alone are in something of the same category. That's one reason diets consistently fail. Instead of bringing you into the stream of life, they set you apart from it—off somewhere with your blender and your portion scale and your food diary. The Love-powered diet, however, recognizes that you are not only a part of life, you are a vital part of it. Love has a vested interest in getting you out of your food rut, because you will be vastly more loving when you are.

Is this going to be complicated? No, it's deceptively simple. Will it be easy? Not all the time, but living the Love-powered way is, at its toughest, easier than trying to convince yourself that the half gallon of ice cream in your shopping cart is for the family, when you know your husband is out of town and both your kids have dairy allergies. Probably the most difficult thing you'll have to grapple with is giving up the fight. You may feel as if you've gone AWOL, but believe me: with Love as your commander-in-chief, you'll be honorably discharged from active combat. You will be able to harmonize an inner awareness of Love with loving outward actions—food choices included.

This harmony is essential for durable change, whether you want to overcome chronic binge-eating, do away with an annoying ten pounds, stop dieting for the first time since puberty, or simply eat a little more healthfully and helpfully than you do now. Life without the dual plagues of compulsive eating and fanatical weight control is precious indeed. Health of body and peace of mind are also priceless commodities. To help you toward these, I offer you the Love-powered diet—if you'd like to change your relationship with food, and you know that willpower is not enough.

-✤✤-

ONE

Food

as a Fix

I was a fat little girl in a fat-phobic family. There was always a diet for me taped to the refrigerator and I only got a milkshake when I was sick. Years later, I had a cold and my boyfriend brought me a French vanilla shake. I married him.

You see, my father had been a physician who'd gradually turned his practice from ear, nose, and throat to fat, flab, and cellulite. My mother managed reducing salons with adipose-jiggling machines and the promise of effortless weight loss. I knew early on that my plumpness was not pleasing and that I was bad for business.

It wasn't that I didn't want to be good and stick to my diet. I knew there were starving children who didn't even have grapefruit and broiled halibut, but the notion of restricting what I ate was terrifying. It meant giving up the sublime security that came from an illicit cookie or carton of ice cream. When I was eating, I felt safe, contented, loved. Once the food was gone, so was the feeling. I needed food to sustain life like everybody else, but I also needed it to face life. I didn't know it then, but I was hooked. Food was my fix.

When I was thirteen, I discovered the flipside of my addiction: the high of being thin. I'd had a severe case of measles and wasn't able to eat for a couple of weeks. Once I got out of bed, I weighed myself: 111 pounds. I had bones. They were wonderful. I was wonderful. I bought a gorgeous green satin dress with puffy sleeves and a dropped waist and flippy little skirt. I was awed by my own reflection in the mirror. Although only 5'5", I looked to myself like the models in the teen magazines. I could have died in peace at that moment: I was finally okay.

I never got to go anywhere in that green satin dress, though. Within the month I was back to 140 pounds and felt for the first time "pitiful and incomprehensible demoralization."[1] That's the phrase the book *Alcoholics Anonymous* uses to describe the state of an alcoholic who had once gained some control and then lost it again. I never drank, but the phrase fit.

A stalwart attempt at controlling my eating came in young adulthood with a popular commercial weight loss system. I followed the recommended diet with religious fervor, refusing to alter it in any way. Even after I reached a goal weight of 120, I stayed on the diet until I weighed in one Saturday morning at ninety-eight pounds. That did it: I had broken the thin barrier. I was cured. I bought a pound of roasted cashews, ate them all on the bus ride home, and gained twenty pounds in forty days. "Pitiful and incomprehensible demoralization" combined with such hatred for my inflated body that I refused to be seen by anyone who knew me. I quit my job and moved to Chicago where I planned to hide, diet, and return at some future date in triumphant thinness.

While in Chicago, I learned to fast, perfecting fourteen-day stints

1. *Alcoholics Anonymous*, p. 8. See Appendix A, "Suggested Reading."

on water only, plus doing several short juice fasts as well. My physical self shrunk obediently every time, but I was so ravenous after each of these Gandhian intervals that I ate enough to go back home in a year and a half with nearly sixty more pounds to my credit. After that, I stayed away from scales.

It took months for my ability to diet to resurface. It was inspired by my boyfriend's taking off for the West Coast, maybe to come back, maybe not. Hurt and anger mobilized my resolve: I would get thin and beautiful and show him what he'd left behind. I lost weight and he proposed, but neither of us realized that I was a food addict, a fact that the size of my body could not alter.

The facade started to crack with little weight gains here and there. They were frightening, and I felt I couldn't trust myself around a refrigerator while subject to any of the ordinary pressures of life— work, my roommate, my cat. The answer: fat farms! I took a week in Texas the first time, then two in Florida. It was becoming an expensive habit, so I started checking myself in at nice local hotels to diet or fast and use their health club facilities. It worked well for a while, but as I needed to go more frequently, cost again became an issue.

I looked for cheaper and cheaper hotels. The last one was a past-its-prime hostelry in the middle of town. The room cost $5. It had a phone book minus the yellow pages and a Gideon Bible lacking most of the New Testament. The carpet had been burned in spots by a careless smoker and the television was chained to the wall. "I'm in a bona fide flophouse," I told myself. "This is skid row and I made my way here with a fork." I cried most of the night because I knew I had become the equivalent of a gutter drunk, but if I told anyone that they'd laugh and tell me to go on a diet.

I knew I was sick and that sick people are supposed to see physicians. I was wary of diet doctors—I'd tried appetite-suppressing shots and pills before and got more wired than wiry. This time I decided to seek the services of a general practitioner who suggested testing me for hypoglycemia (low blood sugar). I took some comfort in the prospect of a genuine diagnosis, especially since so many of the hypoglycemic symptoms sounded like mine: a craving for food, especially sweets, a gripping panic when deprived of food for a long period, along with depression, irritability, and moodiness.

I was scheduled for a six-hour glucose-tolerance test, a grueling ordeal of breaking a twelve-hour fast with a bottle of pure glucose and having blood drawn seven times in the next six hours while taking in no other food. By the end of the test, I thought I'd die. I was nervous, shaky, and dizzy, and would have sold my soul for a turnip. I went straight from the hospital to a convenience store and bought two candy bars, a bag of chips, an ice cream bar, and a diet pop.

When the test results turned out to be normal, I was sure there had been a mistake. I convinced the doctor to arrange for me to be tested whenever I experienced the shakes and lightheadedness that I felt signaled hypoglycemia. I rushed to the lab during a particularly severe episode, expecting to find my blood sugar at some subterranean level. It was normal. After half-a-dozen such forays, I had to accept that the symptoms I was experiencing were not hypoglycemia. They were withdrawal. When I didn't have that comforting sense of fullness, the friendly and accomplished young woman who I often seemed to be gave way to the frightened child who had found comfort in soft white bread and sweet sandwich cookies.

Seeing that kind of emotional connection to food, my next step was to enter counseling. The psychologists I saw pointed out numerous reasons why I ate the way I did. The list was impressive.

1. I'd had a digestive disorder as an infant, so I carried with me a primal fear of starvation.

2. My parents' professions had set me up for an eating disorder. My staying overweight was an unconscious ploy to demand their unconditional love.

3. Since I'd been a fat child, I had a greater number of fat cells than people who were never heavy or who gained weight in adulthood and simply enlarged the fat cells they already had. All those greedy lipid cells were crying out to be fed.

4. I had, according to one unconventional therapist, died of hunger in a former incarnation and was trying to make up for it in this one.

I was grateful to learn all these fascinating hypotheses about my behavior. Unfortunately, being so enlightened didn't change a thing. My physicians had no remedy for my body and my therapists had none for my mind, although I was in need on both counts. The solution, if there was to be one, had to come in another way. And it has. I didn't outgrow my food addiction, I don't have any more willpower than I ever did, and I haven't had broiled halibut in over twenty years. Nevertheless, I didn't eat for a fix today and I didn't obsess over the size and shape of my body. As a practicing food addict, I was helpless, but I was never hopeless. Neither are you.

❦ PATTERNS ❦

You may eat for a fix in many of the ways that I did. The pattern may have started early in life, or when you got married, or after you were divorced. You might trace it to a pregnancy or the loss of someone you loved, or it may have come upon you subtly and gradually. You might eat enormous meals, or snack all day and not even remember when you had your last real breakfast or lunch or dinner. You may only get out of control with chocolates or sugary foods or salty, crunchy things. Perhaps you eat sparingly around people and binge on the sly so no one can understand why you don't lose weight. ("She eats like a bird," you've heard them say, "but she's as big as a horse.")

On the other hand, you may be enviably slim and only you know that you stay that way by throwing up every day, or that your preoccupation with fitness long ago shifted from a healthy habit to a tyrannical compulsion. You could be eating quite reasonably and looking fine but you feel fat, berate yourself, and want to live in a body your heredity didn't provide. Maybe you're so devastated by the addiction that you avoid people as much as you can and hardly bother to wash the one outfit that you can still wear. More likely, though, you seem to function flawlessly and keep on top of everything—except for a little problem with eating. It's also possible that you don't have a serious problem with food or body image at all but it's been six months since your doctor told you to make some changes in your diet to lower your cholesterol or your blood pressure and you haven't been able to do it to save your life.

Whatever category you belong to, you've probably said, "I guess I just like food too much." Well, of course you like food. Everybody does. We're supposed to like it so much that we eat it as long as we live and live as long as we can. That's nature's way. It's only when food seems to choose us instead of our choosing it that something is wrong. **Any time we stuff ourselves, starve ourselves, or eat something we know to be harmful, we're mistreating ourselves. When we do any of these things repeatedly, we establish a self-destructive and self-defeating pattern. When we want to stop and can't, we're addicted.**

Some would argue with that terminology. They would say that food is not a drug that is universally addictive like heroin or even selectively addictive like alcohol. They might argue that food can cause, at worst, a behavioral addiction. The phenomenon of craving, however, exists in food addiction as in any other kind of addiction. I have craved food so strongly that I've taken leftover cake from an office wastebasket, brushed off the cigarette ashes, and eaten all but the cardboard plate. It's been powerful enough to send me out on foot at midnight in search of caramels, and spend a night in a five-dollar hotel room, hoping to escape.

I also know that food can be the object of addiction because I see others and myself recovering by using spiritual principles of transformation. The spiritual approach is also without equal in helping people addicted to other substances and practices. The only real difference in getting over a food addiction as opposed to an addiction to alcohol or cocaine is one of abstemiousness versus abstinence. Alcoholics stop drinking alcohol. Drug addicts stop using mood-altering drugs. Food addicts can't give up eating, but we can stop eating for a fix. **Recovery is a delicate balance somewhere between the binge and the diet. That's where we abandon the struggle and find sanity and peace of mind.**

The dictionary defines recovery as "to get back." For me, it's meant getting back some surprising things. One of them is my youth. I spent so much of my earlier life in the disease that now that I'm past forty, I delight in looking and feeling younger than I am. I'm able to use the nutritional knowledge that I had in abundance (food addicts love learning about food) but could never apply. Those physicians and counselors I'd dismissed as worthless can be helpful now when I consult them for guidance instead of expecting them to provide me with the transformation that had to come from within. I've even been given back the joy of eating. What I did before was drugging, and it was seldom pleasant to my stomach or my conscience. Eating is a pleasure today—that's how it should be—but it's a peripheral pleasure, not the center of my world.

I once hated the way I ate but couldn't change it. The difference started when I gave up willpower for the power of Love—love for myself and from myself, for others and from them, and grounded in the Love that is also Power. I'm comfortable calling that God. You can call it whatever you like. It has, by any name, provided an answer where there seemed to be none, and a life beyond the fix that's filled with hope and humor and expectation. Tapping that Power is essential for addicts to live again, and my hunch is that some of that same Power is needed for almost anyone to make major lifestyle changes that last. If you do not believe in miracles, or if you think they don't happen anymore, just come to my house for dinner.

- - - - - - - - - - - - - - - -

◀ SOME THINGS FOOD ADDICTS MAY DO ▶

- *Hide food*
- *Sneak food*
- *Go on diets—usually on Mondays*
- *Make promises, vows, and deals with themselves, others, and God, about eating less and losing weight*
- *Lie—to themselves, others, and God*
- *Avoid scales or weigh compulsively*
- *Dissociate from their bodies—live from the neck up*
- *Put off living (shopping, swimming, vacationing, sex) until weight is lost*
- *Detest physical exercise—or become addicted to exercise (they may still detest it)*
- *Feel unattractive (or conditionally attractive based upon a scale number or clothing size)*
- *Hate fat people—or hate thin people*

- *Have special binge foods as drugs of choice—chocolate, sweets, and salty snacks are favorites—but could binge on almost anything in a pinch*
- *Eat others' leftovers, unthawed frozen foods, or nonfoods (i.e., wrappers from muffins, used tea bags, chewing gum)*
- *Vomit after a binge or even after a moderate meal or snack (bulimia)*
- *Diet successfully for a time, then fall off and gain back as much or more weight than was lost (ability to diet eventually ceases altogether)*
- *Fast at times relatively easily, finding it less trying to eat nothing than to eat moderately*
- *Feed other people, especially when they're depriving themselves*
- *Cook and bake—although in later stages of the disease these may fall aside in favor of readymade, instant gratification items*
- *Please people, be "sweet"*
- *Deal inappropriately with anger—either denying ("stuffing") it or having attacks of rage, usually toward someone powerless, i.e., a child or pet*
- *Switch compulsions, e.g., giving up food for a time and becoming addicted to drugs (i.e., diet pills), relationships, or spending*

❄ SOME THINGS FOOD ADDICTS MAY THINK ❄

- *This (diet, pill, doctor) will be the one that works.*
- *I ate too much (or gained weight) so I'm a bad person.*
- *No one else eats like I do.*
- *If you really knew me, you wouldn't like me.*
- *I'm fat and disgusting.*
- *I broke my diet so I'm a failure.*
- *I ate two extra peas. That means I've blown it and have to eat half a gallon of ice cream.*
- *I've lost weight now and life is supposed to be perfect.*

- *I've lost weight now so I'm cured.*
- *This time I'll just have a little bit.*
- *I'll get back on my diet tomorrow.*
- *Eating will make me feel better.*
- *I have to eat something to get through this . . . (tragedy, term paper, telephone call).*
- *When I lose weight, I'll be beautiful.*
- *When I lose weight, my husband/wife/lover will love me (or I'll get a husband/wife/lover who will love me).*
- *When I lose weight, my mother/father/other significant childhood figure will love and accept me (even if they're dead).*
- *When I lose weight, I'll do everything I ever wanted to do.*
- *I feel fat (in response to being full, premenstrual, or constipated, also in response to rejection, disappointment, or presumed failure).*
- *If I eat while I read it won't count (the same goes for food sampled during cooking).*
- *I deserve to treat myself (with food) and I deserve to punish myself (also with food).*

. . . .

❧ SOME THINGS PEOPLE SAY TO FOOD ADDICTS ❧ (THAT DON'T HELP AT ALL)

- *Use a little willpower.*
- *Push yourself away from the table.*
- *I've got this great diet for you.*
- *Just eat less.*
- *How could you let yourself get this way?*
- *I need to be perfectly honest with you . . . (followed by almost anything).*
- *You have such a pretty face.*
- *I remember when you wore a size five (or eight or ten).*

- *Your sister/brother/friend trimmed down so nicely.*
- *I'll come over at six tomorrow and we'll jog.*
- *C'mon, you gotta shape up if you want to attract the ladies (or men).*
- *I don't know how to tell you this, but do you realize you have a weight problem?*
- *You really look perfectly fine—well, except you could lose a few pounds.*
- *You're too old to change how you eat (versus You're too young not to).*
- *I'm only concerned about your health.*
- *You know, gluttony is a sin.*
- *Take one of these pills whenever you get hungry.*
- *Beauty is only skin deep anyhow.*
- *Do what I did and put a sign on your refrigerator that says, 'Oink!'*
- *You can have just one! (Variation: A little won't hurt this once.)*
- *I made this especially for you.*
- *You'd feel so much better about yourself if you lost a little weight.*
- *I clipped out this article about how being overweight shortens life expectancy.*
- *I lost five lbs. taking these great vitamins—in fact, I'm selling them now.*
- *You just need to get ahold of yourself (with or without an addendum about how much of oneself there is to get ahold of).*

—✦✦—

TWO

The Body

and the

Spirit

Like stepchildren in fairy tales, our bodies get blamed for a lot. When we criticize them, we put ourselves down, too. If you've ever said, "I hate my thighs," or "I used to be pretty but now I'm a wreck," or "Look at this fat—I'm really disgusting!", you've been your own evil stepmother.

Your weight may be a problem, but it isn't *the* problem. It's a symptom—usually a symptom of out-of-control eating. You can be rid of the symptom while the real problem flourishes. Getting thin is not a cure. Any size six bulimic can attest to that. Nevertheless, if you deal with the *cause* of the overweight, your body will reflect a wellness, a balance, and a beauty that go far beyond how you look in a pair of shorts.

INNER MALAISE ⟶ DESTRUCTIVE EATING ⟶ OVERWEIGHT

The little flow chart above should help explain it. We have a continuum here. It starts with what I'm calling inner malaise. That's a catchall term to cover the fear and discontent, stress and impaired self-image, childhood leftovers or anything else that stands between us and our being at peace with ourselves and our world. Inner malaise can lead to a variety of inappropriate or self-destructive behaviors. Destructive eating is the one we're concerned with here. It generally shows up as extra weight.

Traditionally, we've gone after the obvious: the weight. And why not? We can see it. We can even weigh it, for heaven's sake! But when it's gone (via diets, exercise, pills, you name it), the inner malaise can still be active, resulting in further destructive eating. In fact, as long as the inner malaise goes unchecked, even dieting is destructive eating (or destructive noneating). It will eventually lead to gaining back the lost weight, or to some variation on the theme, such as bulimia.

This is not to say that there are no physical reasons for overweight. There are several. Refined sugars and greasy, salty snacks actually cause an addictive reaction in some people and lead to overeating (you'll read more about this in Chapter 6 when we discuss binge foods). Too much fat in the diet can result in too much fat on the body, and lack of exercise can lower the metabolic rate, encouraging fat storage. Dieting is also a factor: "The body cannot distinguish dieting from starvation. . . . We are automatically driven to gorge ourselves in anticipation of recurrent famine."[1]

These physical phenomena have become widely known in recent years. Knowing about them and doing something about them are obviously two very different things. What is it that keeps people from doing what they know would bring them what they want? For a great

---

1. Neal D. Barnard, M.D., *The Power of Your Plate*, p. 88. This "restrained eater phenomenon" is detailed by Dr. Barnard in his chapter, "New Strategies for Weight Control." See Appendix A, "Suggested Reading."

many people—and only you can decide if you're one of them—inner malaise blocks their attempt to put into practice the good things they already know about nutrition and a healthy lifestyle.

Some people have realized that attacking the weight is a hopeless maneuver and they have proposed alternative plans of action that focus on the middle of the chart, the eating itself. Their strategy is generally behavior modification—techniques such as taking small bites and putting the fork down between them, or forgoing the fork altogether and giving chopsticks a try. The idea is to shut out old habits with new ones, like not eating alone or after seven in the evening. These can be positive practices, but most of the time they fail over the long haul. Why? They fail because our actions ultimately grow out of ourselves. Unless we change, our actions are not likely to change.

On the other hand, when the inner malaise itself is addressed, both the harmful eating patterns *and* the resultant overweight lose their source and sustenance. Tiny miracles transpire one by one. We take those smaller bites. We aren't hanging on to the fork as if it were a life preserver. Breathing gets easier. Clothes get looser. And although we never asked for this one, *life gets better*. It has to, because it is being lived in a new and decidedly better way.

◄ HEALING AT THE DESIRE LEVEL ►

When the healing comes like this, from within, it's healing at the desire level. It's no longer wanting a candy bar and settling for an orange. It's wanting the orange and relishing every bite of it. This does not mean that there will never again be food choices to make. There are healthful and unhealthful food choices just as there are healthful and unhealthful life choices. Only by dealing with the inner malaise, though, are we able to truly make choices about what we eat. Otherwise, the choices are made for us, and we usually regret them.

When we turn to unhealthful or excessive food (or any other damaging substance or practice) in order to feel better, it's because something is missing in our lives. Although it seems that what we lack is outside ourselves—the right job, the right mate, the right body, the right memories—the emptiness is core-deep. **To make satisfying, lasting changes in how we nourish our bodies requires that we** learn to get some vital nourishment from within. **We do that by connecting with our spiritual selves, by making practical contact with the Divine, whatever we perceive that to be.**

Words like "spiritual" and "Divine" (capitalized, no less!) can be loaded with emotional definitions that aren't likely to show up in the dictionary, but which can vividly color our personal interpretations. It may be that you're not a religious person and you've got me pegged as a holy roller. Or perhaps you are religious and you wonder if I'm from some cult that collects money in airports. I'm neither (honest!), but what's important to get you free from the food fix is not what I am but what you are.

If you can get past the binge/diet syndrome by some other means, terrific. I couldn't. I'd stressed my resolve and my willpower until, like overworked peasants, they chose to revolt. That insidious urge to smooth life's rough edges with a nibble that could turn into a nightmare would overtake me just when I was convinced that I had everything under control. My intelligence and good intentions were of no more use than lighting fixtures in a house with no wiring. I needed power and I didn't have it. I needed to tap into a Higher Power, one that would always be there.

It was such a strange notion. My problem had seemed so *physical*. I ate quantities of physical food and it showed quantitatively on my physical body, yet paradoxically the answer to my problem was spiritual. It didn't make sense to me at first, and it may not make sense to you until you realize that, as human beings, you and I are like icebergs. What people see, our physical selves, is only the tip of who we are. There's lots more beneath the surface. We're splendid beings with complex emotions and intellects, and underlying our hearts, minds, and bodies is a spiritual essence. It is uniquely ours, yet it connects us to every living thing. It connects us to Life itself.

The part of you that shows, your body, *is* important because it is a part of you and *you* are important. You can think of your body as the vehicle by which you journey through this life, as your radio receiver for picking up the signals of the outside world, or as an instrument in an orchestra, allowing you to play your music for the rest of us. A symphony needs French horns and oboes, cellos and violins, tinkling little triangles, and booming bass drums. You might even be a grand piano!

Abusing food can interfere with your ability to appreciate your special physical self. In an all-out binge, it's necessary to, in effect, cut off diplomatic relations between the body and the mind. Since it's a rare person who consciously *wants* to be miserable, most people who binge separate their conscious (thinking) selves from their sensory (physical) selves by reading, working, driving, or watching television while they eat. They may absentmindedly grab snacks throughout the day or tastes while cooking a meal. Swearing off the distractions that remove you from the present moment may seem like the antidote, but it isn't. If you have the *need* to binge, you will find a way to shut off your mind—with all its "shoulds" and "oughts" and "know betters"—and go for the food.

The need to binge is a spiritual hunger. It can only be assuaged with spiritual food. You know how koala bears eat nothing but eucalyptus leaves? The soul is something like that. It can only be nourished by Love. (There's that capital again.) You see, all genuine love is good—love from your family, your friends, even your companion animals—but the kind you need for this purpose can't be filtered through anyone else. It has to be from the Source: Love that's within you so you don't have to look for it, that's already yours so you don't have to earn it, that can't stop loving so you needn't worry about losing it.

I think that was the kind Rilke was referring to when he wrote in *Letters to a Young Poet,* " . . . believe in a love that is being held for you like an inheritance and trust that in this love there is a strength and a blessing, out beyond which you do not have to step in order to go very far!"[2] That inheritance is yours. You claim it first by wanting it. Once you do, you'll be eager to put into practice the principles you'll learn in this book. The first are these:

1. Accept that your food problem is serious, that you can't deal with it on your own.

2. Open your mind to the idea that a Higher Power can help.

3. Allow that Power—call it Love, call it God, call it whatever feels absolutely right to you—to work some wonders in your life.

If you're familiar with the Twelve Steps of Alcoholics Anonymous, adopted by Overeaters Anonymous, Gamblers Anonymous, Co-

2. Rainer Maria Rilke, *Letters To A Young Poet*, translation by M. D. Herter Norton (New York: W. W. Norton & Co., Inc., rev. ed., 1954), p. 40.

dependents Anonymous, and numerous other groups, you'll recognize these three concepts as an interpretation of the first three Steps.[3] People in the Anonymous programs sometimes abbreviate these Steps as, "I can't, God can, I'll let Him (or Her or It)." However worded, this formula is common to men and women of all ages and cultures who have built, or rebuilt, their lives on a spiritual basis, letting go of old ways that didn't work and inviting in something that does.

◀❧ A LIFETIME ADVENTURE ❧▶

Spiritualizing your thoughts and attitudes is an adventure that can last a lifetime. To instigate the process, particularly as it affects your eating, take the following actions today and every day for the next month.

1. Each morning before your feet touch the floor, ask your Higher Power to help you eat reasonably that day, and say thank you at night even if your eating didn't seem perfect.

2. When you get to a mirror to wash your face or shave, look yourself in the eye and say, "I love you just the way you are." You don't have to believe it, just do it.

3. Read over the "Revolutionary Concepts" beginning on page 25 morning and evening.

4. Get some quiet time to yourself every single day—at least ten minutes' worth. If you have to take this time in the bathtub to get privacy, fine. During your quiet minutes, read over the first three of the Twelve Steps (Appendix D) and think about them. Do you really believe that you're powerless over your addiction or is there something else you'd like to try? Can you contemplate the possibility that a Higher Power could help? Can you consider making a decision to put that Higher Power in charge of your will and your life? (Writing your thoughts on this in a journal isn't required, but it can be helpful.)

5. *Do not diet.* Think instead in terms of not eating for a fix *one day at a time*. Get three reasonable meals every day and before each one ask your Higher Power to help you eat wisely. If you want to eat

---

3. The Twelve Steps are listed in full in Appendix D.

between meals, converse with your Higher Power. If you're really hungry, have a piece of fruit.

6. Do two nice things for yourself today—one that you think you "should" (make the bed, floss your teeth, swim laps), and one that's just for fun (take a bubble bath, rent a video, call a friend long-distance). Don't be surprised if it's easier to enjoy the work than the play.

7. Enlist some support. At the very least, read this book with a friend and then help each other along. You'll do yourself a far greater favor if you hook up with a support group already organized that uses proven principles to help food addicts recover. I recommend Overeaters Anonymous. OA will teach you to incorporate the Twelve Steps into your life while providing an unparalleled support system of people who understand. OA meetings are in every major city and most smaller ones, and there is no charge for membership. (For more information, see the listing for Overeaters Anonymous in Appendix C, "Some Helpful Organizations.")

If you're feeling overwhelmed by all this, relax. You're not in a competition and you don't have to pass a quiz. Many of the ideas you have just read are probably new to you. Give yourself time to let them settle, and feel free to read this chapter more than once before you go further. You're embarking on a transformational journey. That's no small thing. It's certainly understandable if you're feeling some trepidation. There is a lot at stake here. Old patterns of doing things are going to be replaced. They don't want to get fired.

While you're making layoffs, you may also want to consider trading any old images of a punishing, wrathful deity for a Higher Power that loves you no matter what. You'll need one that isn't just interested in great, cosmic events but one that's interested in you and seeing you out of your food addiction. The image I like is that if God were the sun, each and every one of us would get our own personal beam, keeping us safe and warm. You can use any image that speaks to you. Just get used to being loved unconditionally. Before long, you'll be loving yourself unconditionally, too. (Unconditional, you know, includes thighs.)

And you are not only lovable. You are also, whether you realize it or not, spiritual. Do not think for an instant that because the solution to food addiction is spiritual, food addicts themselves somehow aren't. **In the midst of a binge, anyone's spirituality is on temporary hold, but your inherent spiritual identity persists. Being overweight, bulimic, or in some other way obsessed with food or with your body does not negate that identity.**

All the inner growth you've done up to this point counts, too. Only you and God know how far you've had to come to get here, to the point where you can look honestly at yourself and what you are eating. Give yourself some credit, and resist the urge to compare yourself to anyone else. Many people have never had a serious problem with food. Others have overcome food addictions while you were growing through something else. All that matters now is that you've suffered with this long enough. It's your turn to be free—body and spirit.

- - - - - - - - - - - - - - - - -

◄ PHASE OUT FAT DAYS ►

Do you ever have fat days? On fat days you feel fat regardless of your size. These days can be precipitated by eating too much, a little too much, or just what you think is too much. They can also be brought on by such seeming irrelevancies as having dirty hair or an argument with someone who's important in your life. Losing weight isn't a fully satisfactory response to fat days since they're so subjective. As an extreme but telling example, think of anorexics. I've visited some in hospitals who were painfully, even frighteningly, emaciated, yet who felt fat. For them, every day was a fat day, although they had literally been in danger of dying from malnutrition.

While anorexia is a psychiatric disorder that requires professional help, seeing the body in a distorted way is so common that it's generally accepted as the way things are. But what if instead of fat days you had poison ivy days, when you itched all over even though there was nothing organically wrong? It would seem like a problem, wouldn't it? Well, fat days are a problem, too, because they're days on which you tend to love yourself less than you deserve. You are lovable every day. You can't force yourself to believe that, but you can allow for the possibility that it's true to enter your world view. Allowing for such possibilities is a spiritual activity because it happens deep within you.

A long time ago a friend said to me, "When I'm 150 pounds going up, I'm the fattest, ugliest person on earth, but when I'm 150 coming down, I'm absolutely beautiful." In the years since she made that statement, my friend has done a lot of inner work to realize that she's beautiful all the time. It so happens that she hasn't had an eating binge in a dozen years, so the whole notion of "going up" and "coming down" only touches her life today as it relates to elevators and airplane trips.

Spiritual recovery means more than an end to eating for a fix. It also implies befriending your body. You don't wait to do that until after you've reached some arbitrary goal weight. You do it today, the first day that you put your food choices in the hands of a loving Higher Power. The imaging ability of the mind that can be twisted to give you fat days can be uplifted to give you attractive and healthy days. As these days go by, your physical body will catch up with your mental image. Since the body is subject to physical laws, it will take some time for its form to change, but the time it takes for you to be happy and to have an attractive, healthy day is no time at all. Enjoy it.

⚜ REVOLUTIONARY CONCEPTS ⚜

These revolutionary concepts aren't for taking over embassies, they're the beginners' basics for revolutionizing your relationship with your body and how you feed it. Read them over morning and evening for thirty days, paying particular attention to those with which you may feel uncomfortable. It's possible that those won't apply to you at all, but it's more likely that they're precisely the ones that can mean the most in your recovery.

You are acceptable right now, regardless of what you ate yesterday or what the scale has to say about you.

·

Abusing food is a sign of internal imbalance, and overcoming it is largely an inside job.

Food addiction is serious and, like other addictions, progressive. Few genuine addicts have ever recovered without a spiritual basis.

·

Your spirituality is personal. You don't have to take on someone else's brand.

·

You are a spiritual being living in a physical body. Your body is an integral part of the totality that is you.

·

Your body is not an independent entity; it reflects what's going on inside you—emotionally, mentally, and spiritually.

·

It's okay to feel beautiful right now. If you wait until you're thin to feel beautiful, you may never get there.

·

If you don't eat for a fix today, that long string of tomorrows that seems so foreboding will take care of itself.

·

Your body is not your enemy. You are in this together. When you do something nice for your body, you're doing something nice for yourself.

·

Having a food addiction does not make you a bad person. Both medicine and psychology recognize addiction as an illness, not a moral issue.

·

You don't have to be perfect to get well, and it's even all right to be a little bit scared.

·

Ideas you're not sure of can be tried out, like taking a car on a test drive. If, for example, the thought of a spiritual solution to your food problem doesn't seem logical, you can consider it a possibility, a working hypothesis.

—❈❈—

THREE

Getting to

Point Zero

A race is only fair if every contestant starts at the starting line. If life were a race, though, some of us would have to run a veritable marathon just to get to the place where everyone else seems fresh and rested, eager to take off. I call that place *Point Zero*. At Point Zero, you're free, unencumbered, and your chances for winning are as good as anybody's. Eating for a fix, however, can keep you from getting there.

Healthy people meet every new day, every new dilemma, every new project from the level ground of Point Zero. Because they like themselves, they're comfortable with life and aren't likely to become addicted to anything. They're not perfect and don't need to be, but they're at home in their own skins and in the world around them. When they have difficulties, they're able to get the help they need and use the help they get, whether it comes from friends, family, professionals, or their own inner resources. They rebound well from adversity and although they may lose many things in life, hope won't be one of them. At Point Zero, there is always hope, spirited challenge, and limitless potential.

Addictive behavior keeps Point Zero elusive. Food addicts now in recovery have described it in these ways:

> I felt like I was in an invisible box and couldn't get out. People kept offering me advice and ideas that I couldn't use because I couldn't get out of the box to try them. I see now that I'd built the box myself and that I'd built it with a tight-fitting lid.

> There was one awful thing in my life: the way I ate. I was really angry that I couldn't do anything about it since I seemed to be so good at everything else. It seemed like a terrible blight to me, a stigma.

> My life looked great: I was busy all the time but when I was alone something always seemed to be missing. It was "quiet desperation." I acted happy—you know, "jolly"—but I was so sad.

As you can see from the following diagram, Point Zero is sort of an alchemical crossroad at which the old baggage of subzero attitudes and actions is turned into golden qualities. Obsessive eating no longer fits. You accept life on life's terms. You're a participant in it, not a spectator. Fear is transmuted into safe, healing, conditionless Love. It provides the foundation for the best possible relationships with yourself, other people, and the myriad things that make up your life—your work, your interests, your finances, your food. When you clear away what stands between you and Point Zero, you will be able to tap into that Love, which has always been available, more easily than ever before. Once you do, you'll find yourself showing up when life is passing the good stuff your way, and when circumstances aren't the best, you won't be brought down with them.

The fear-motivated thought and action patterns you see on the diagram beneath the zero point lead away from self-love and self-care. It

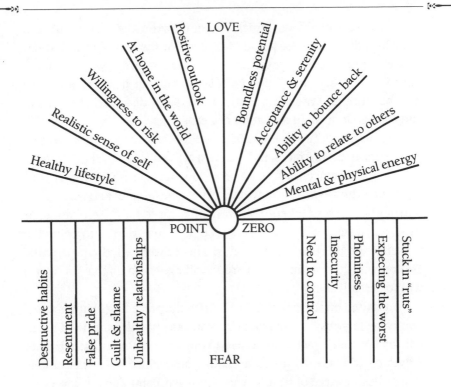

LOVE

Positive outlook
At home in the world
Willingness to risk
Realistic sense of self
Healthy lifestyle

Boundless potential
Acceptance & serenity
Ability to bounce back
Ability to relate to others
Mental & physical energy

POINT ZERO

Destructive habits
Resentment
False pride
Guilt & shame
Unhealthy relationships

Need to control
Insecurity
Phoniness
Expecting the worst
Stuck in "ruts"

FEAR

doesn't make you a bad person to be acquainted with those patterns; they are simply thoughts and actions that do not work to bring you what you want in life. They worked at one time or you wouldn't have developed them. They were protection mechanisms that were once useful, but which have come to do more harm than good—like an old pair of glasses that used to help you see better but now make everything a blur. The glasses served their purpose, but it's time for a new prescription.

Using food (or extra weight) as a buffer between yourself and life is one way to keep old patterns intact and stay negative, in the red, below Point Zero. This does not mean that because you and I have histories of misusing food that we are or ever were less than the next person. The very fact that we're alive makes us remarkable. Besides, you can come from a respected family, be highly intelligent, well-educated, and gainfully employed but still feel subzero inside.

It might manifest as feeling out of place much of the time, or as if you're somehow different from other people. You may be tired from trying to catch up to some invisible goal or meet some impossible standard. You might recognize as your own some of the subzero thinking patterns in "A Mental Makeover" at the end of this chapter. However much or little you relate to these examples, if you're still using food in a way you're uncomfortable with (or if you're not right now but are afraid you will again), there is some distance between you and the freedom you'll find at Point Zero.

The mission at hand, then, is to get to Point Zero from wherever you're starting. In one sense, there isn't far to go—about twelve inches, the distance from your head to your heart. In terms of consciousness, however, this may be the most meaningful and fascinating journey you've ever taken. You won't make it to Point Zero alone, or by sheer effort or willpower. You need to resign yourself to being the passenger on this trip: Love (God, Higher Power) will do the driving. You only need to get in the car. Your willingness to do that uses your will to best advantage.

You started on the trek to Point Zero in the preceding chapter when you came to grips with the fact that you can't handle your food problem by yourself, when you allowed yourself to believe that a Higher Power could make the difference, and you decided to let that Loving Power be in charge of things. You will reach Point Zero as you clean up the past and learn to live fearlessly and productively in the present. For your part in this process you must:

- Become more honest than you've ever been
- Become willing to postpone eating for a fix
- Learn to sit with your feelings
- Make peace with the past and with people
- Expand your comfort zone

Underlying all of these are spiritual verities which have shown themselves over time to make people's lives better. Because truth is well told in fable, I will introduce each one of the five ways for getting to Point Zero with a story.

Becoming More Honest

There was once a shaman whose fame for miraculous healings spread far and wide. The people of his country were astounded by the miracles he per-

formed and discoursed among themselves about how he accomplished them. "He becomes as tiny as a gnat," one suggested, "and goes into the sick body, sees what is wrong and eats it away." "No," argued another, "he becomes as tall as the sky and lifts the sick person up to the gods. It is they that do the magic." The shaman overheard this conversation and gently interrupted: "I am no larger or smaller than either of you, my friends. And the healings you see are not magic. I have simply spoken the truth in earnestness for such a long time that my words cannot be false. When I say someone is well, he can be nothing else."

Honesty is not optional if you want to live without a food problem. *The Answer to Addiction*, a marvelous book by three recovered alcoholics on overcoming all sorts of addictions, explains it this way: "You connect with God by means of the truth. And you connect with the truth by stopping lying."[1]

Most of us don't think of ourselves as overt liars, but a solid commitment to honesty is such a rarity that borderline dishonesty passes as acceptable and even commendable. It's usually little things—a waiter forgets to charge for dessert and the customer ignores it, or a six-year-old is passed off as five to get free admission to a theme park or a free ride on the bus. The individual incidents don't amount to much, but they reflect a pervasive lack of regard for honesty in general. It wasn't long ago that "I give you my word" was as good as collateral, but that's no longer the case. The result is that it takes a lot for people to trust one another. Even worse is the fact that we're often not sure we can trust ourselves.

Addiction breeds dishonesty, usually in subtle ways: "I really didn't eat much dinner" (but you finished off all the leftovers), "I just didn't like anything I tried on" (nothing fit), or "I think I'll stay in tonight and get some work done" (being home alone is a great way to binge in peace). To become more honest—even if you believe that you're as honest as you need to be already—*The Answer to Addiction* offers the following suggestions:

As a starter, stop lying to yourself about your addicted condition. . . . Next, stop lying to get out of jams or to smooth off the rough edges of life. Don't lie for the sake of peace; don't lie when common sense invites

1. John Burns, et al., *The Answer to Addiction*, p. 47. See Appendix A, "Suggested Reading."

you to do so; don't lie to cover up your past; don't lie on job applications, expense accounts or tax returns; don't lie to your boss; don't lie to your husband or wife. Just don't lie. When you fail in this resolve (as you will) admit it promptly. And don't indulge failure; that is, don't fail any oftener than you have to.[2]

An excellent place to initiate a commitment to honesty—although probably the most frightening—is as it concerns your eating. First, be honest with yourself about what you're putting in your mouth. Just because you eat something quickly and get rid of the wrapper, or because there isn't anyone else around, doesn't mean you didn't eat it. Did you really have "a few potato chips" or was it three bags? If it was three bags, acknowledge that it was three bags. Denying reality doesn't change it, but dishonesty brings on dangerous rationalization: "I just had a few so it won't make any difference if I have a few more."

While you're at it, it won't hurt to be honest about your weight. In a lot of ways, weight is a silly measurement of anything. It can fluctuate from day to day and scales vary in their readings, but let's face it: you know just about how much you weigh. If you have to renew your driver's license, how awful would it be to tell the truth? Maybe it would be awful, but the perks you get back from telling the truth *about everything* are incredible. You deserve them.

Being truthful will hasten your progress toward freedom from the food fix more assuredly than any other single action. When your personal code of ethics includes both *accepting* the truth and *speaking* the truth, you'll see remarkable improvements in your life. Try me on this one: commit yourself to a *totally* honest day and see how much easier it is to eat reasonably. I'd also wager that you'll go to sleep that night with a particularly peaceful feeling.

Your experiment with expanded honesty will be helped tremendously if there are people around you whom you can trust with honest confidences. These may be the ones who are closest to you, although sometimes it can be more difficult to be up front with significant others than with anyone else. Connecting with other food addicts who are committed to recovery can be a real blessing in this regard. If nothing else, be sure that there is one other person in this world with

2. *The Answer to Addiction*, p. 47.

whom you are willing to be absolutely honest, and share with him or her on a regular basis.

In time, dishonesty simply won't feel comfortable in any circumstances. This doesn't mean that you'll become harsh toward other people. "Honest to a fault" has been used to describe those who like to criticize. With honesty based on Love, however, you'll be able to speak kindly *and* truthfully. You will also know when it's best to say nothing at all. This sort of intuition comes about as a result of your commitment to the truth. As that commitment grows, your true self—the one that's at Point Zero, healthy, happy and addiction-free—will start to emerge as well.

Postponing the Fix

A severe storm destroyed all the huts in a small village. In the days that followed, the villagers were hard at work reconstructing their dwellings before the next rain. One man alone sat at the site where his hut had been, gathering no building materials and lifting no tools. "Why are you not building a shelter?" his neighbors queried. "The rains will come again soon." The man was unmoved. "God took my house from me. He owes me another. I am waiting for God to build it." It was not long before rains again poured down upon the village. The homeless man beat on the doors of his neighbors who thought him lazy and would not let him in. He disappeared into the forest. Some believe he perished, but the wise tell their children how the man lost his senses in the woodland and lives there yet, wild and half-starved, his home the branches of a tree. "That," they warn the children, "is the best house you can expect if you refuse to give God a helping hand."

You can offer that helping hand with your willingness to postpone the fix. The Love-powered diet will become your way of life as you live by Love-powered principles. In that way, it's a gift. You accept the gift every time you refrain from using food for the wrong reasons. It may seem paradoxical to suggest that you do so since the first step in recovery was the admission that you *couldn't* control your eating. That surrender, however, implied a transfer of power: you traded personal power for Love's power, God's power. Therefore, even if you think you cannot possibly do it, you will be able to postpone eating for a fix.

Recovering addicts of all stripes have used the twenty-four-hour plan first recommended by Alcoholics Anonymous. For alcoholics, it means not picking up the first drink, the only one that matters, during a single twenty-four-hour period, this one. In dealing with other compulsions, it means not popping the first pill, placing the first bet, lighting the first cigarette, or in this case, swallowing the first inappropriate mouthful.

We're not able to say, "Starting this Monday I'm going on 1,200 calories until I've lost twenty-five pounds." We've done that and sooner or later it's always backfired. What we are able to do is refrain from inappropriate eating today, just this day, from the time we awaken in the morning until we go to sleep at night.[3] Neither yesterday nor tomorrow has any place in practicing a new way of life. It can only be done in the immediacy of the present, living in what Dr. Maxwell Maltz called in *Psycho-Cybernetics* "daytight compartments."[4]

As you work with the spiritual ideas presented here, your impulses to use food in unhealthful ways will diminish. Eventually, only in rare incidences will the urge to turn to food surface. When it does, you'll actually appreciate it as a signal that something isn't right inside. By then you'll have ample tools for inner growth and hopefully a supportive community as well. With these, you can learn what you need from the feelings you're experiencing, long before they lead you to the refrigerator or the deli.

In the beginning, however, you may have the desire to eat inappropriately rather often. Inappropriate eating includes situations like these:

· It's eleven in the morning. You're at the office. The boss has told you to redo a report you've worked on all week. Lunch isn't for another hour, but as you look around you think you could eat this morning's mail, your Rolodex, and a fax machine.

---

3. Some people are night eaters who get out of bed to raid the icebox. At times they don't even remember the nocturnal foray until they get to the kitchen the next morning and find the evidence. This can be a difficult problem and often professional help is a valuable adjunct in the recovery process. Nevertheless, the use of proven spiritual principles has relieved all sorts of problem eaters, even the after-hours variety. If you are a night eater, I especially urge you to give up going it alone and seek out a recovery group such as Overeaters Anonymous.
4. Maxwell Maltz, M.D., *Psycho-Cybernetics* (New York, Pocket Books, 1986).

- You're in bed with a cold. You just had a substantial lunch but it didn't taste like anything. Besides, there's nobody around to take care of you. A little something would really help—you know, a little sweet thing or a little salty thing.

- You've stopped smoking, but you miss the pleasant prolonging of dinner a cigarette used to provide. Lately you've substituted with extra helpings and second desserts.

- There's no avoiding it: this is cleaning day. You had breakfast and you've descended on the bathrooms. You're fine on the basins and tubs, but then comes the floors. You hate doing floors. This seems like an ideal time for a snack.

- Your son's music lesson lasts an hour. It's not mealtime and you're not really hungry, but the only thing you can think of to do with the time between dropping him off and picking him up is to go somewhere for a bite.

- Your spouse brought in some cookies last night. They're the good ones. You know in your heart of hearts that eating one means eating the package, but you do it anyway.

Remember that as Love-powered living becomes a habit, these very situations can present themselves and you will almost never have the urge to respond to them with eating. When you do, the technique of postponement will prove invaluable. Start with a twenty-four-hour solution. This is the day you're concerned about. You may need to shorten the time frame, be willing to put off the fix for two hours, or one, or fifteen minutes.

And what good does that do? Plenty. For one thing, if you've just finished a meal and want more, it may simply reflect physiological lag time. It takes about twenty minutes for the satiation center in the brain to register that you are full. When you allow that period of time to elapse, your desire to continue eating may abate and you will need to do nothing else. In addition, you can use that postponement time to get yourself centered. This is particularly important if you want to eat for emotional rather than physical reasons—even if you can't at the time tell one from the other.

Centering means finding that point of peace within yourself. It is there. It's there now, even if you're holding this book in your right hand and a candy bar in your left. It's there when you're on the giving or receiving end of an angry outburst, or when you're in turmoil over making a decision and having any peace inside you at all seems like a fantastic notion. At that centered place you can most easily connect with the power of Love that will do for you what food never could. There are a variety of calming techniques such as relaxation and meditation (see Chapter 4, "Looking In, Reaching Out,") to bring you to this state of mind. Prayer or meditation at the time you want to open the refrigerator door can be of real help, providing you truly *want* the help you ask for. Preventive prayer—making a routine of daily quiet time—can fill empty places in advance so you won't look to whatever is in the fridge to do it.

In addition to meditation and prayer, you can go from frantic to stable by engaging in any nondestructive activity that you enjoy. It's a smart move to make a list of the feel-good things you like to do, because if you wait until you want to eat everything that can't run faster than you, the only feel-good thing you'll be able to remember is eating. Photocopy your list and place one in several key spots: your bedside table, your desk at home and at the office, your car, and of course somewhere in the kitchen. Your list will be your own. Mine looks like this:

Happy Stuff
1. Quality time with my daughter, especially reading aloud
2. Organizing some small space in my life, maybe a drawer or a closet
3. Comedy, even on T.V.
4. Brushing our cats
5. Going to a movie, especially those victory-of-the-human-spirit types
6. A hot bath
7. A circuit at the gym
8. Delicious music—the Pachelbel Canon, anything by Mozart

9. Stimulating conversation with someone whose company delights me

10. Making contact with nature—seeing a deer, feeding squirrels in the yard or pigeons in the park, reading or writing in a pretty, natural spot

My list is actually longer than this. Happiness lists tend to grow as your awareness of the many pleasant things in life broadens. Obviously, the desire to eat inappropriately can strike when you aren't free to hop in the bathtub or take a book to the woods. Then you need immediate postponement techniques that also connect you with your spiritual Source. Among them are:

· Read a paragraph or two of something helpful—this book or one of those in Appendix A.

· Call someone you know to be supportive of your desire to eat rationally.

· Change your environment, even for a few minutes, i.e., using your coffee break at work to get outside, walk around a little, breathe some fresher air.

· Write down how you're feeling. You may be surprised by what comes out. Putting emotions and confusions down in black and white can be both revealing and freeing. You might think of it as praying on paper.

· Get by yourself for a couple of minutes, even it it's in the washroom, and have a mini-quiet-time. Ask your Higher Power to help you get through the craving until it passes.

There is no such thing as a craving that doesn't wear itself out. Most people never realize that. They either give in to the craving as soon as it surfaces, or fight it and end up exhausted. They can't see that cravings usually exit before long if they're denied attention.[5]

Another effective postponement technique is also significant in getting to Point Zero. That is learning to sit with your feelings.

---

5. Overeaters Anonymous has excellent literature that addresses "the first compulsive bite." Useful pamphlets include "A Commitment to Abstinence," "Before You Take That First Compulsive Bite," and "The Tools of Recovery."

Sitting with Feelings

Long ago there lived a woman who believed her house to be possessed by demons. She called on the local priest to exorcise them. The priest performed the proper rites, but within a week the woman was again at the rectory gate. "My house is once more possessed!" she cried. The priest performed the ritual a second time and instructed his parishioner to return home.

Not a day had passed before the woman beseeched him a third time to cleanse her house. This request the good father refused. "The terrors that alarm you," he told her, "are less within the walls of your house than within those of your mind. You must confront these spirits yourself."

"But won't you give me something to help—a vial of holy water, a sacred crucifix?" the woman pleaded. "I will give you something," the priest replied. "I will give you a holy stool." He took from the corner a simple wooden hassock. It didn't look particularly holy, but the woman took it none the less. When she entered her house, demons abounded from cellar to loft. "I am lost," she thought. "Even with this holy stool as a weapon, I could never fight them all." She sat on the stool to await her fate, but the instant she was comfortably seated the demons disappeared.

The woman was convinced from that day forward that the cleric's gift indeed bore divine power. The priest, however, knew that her demons departed simply because she had been willing to sit with them. And he missed his favorite footstool for the rest of his life.

For all our contemporary sophistication, many of us are terrified by demons. The ones we fear are not supernatural, they're our own feelings. We label some as negative—grief, remorse, anger, wounded pride—and feel justified in avoiding contact with them. Sometimes, however, we're equally uncomfortable with positive emotions. We're cautious about accepting compliments (we may not deserve them), feeling too good (we might jinx it), or even loving someone (they could go away). A tried and true way to keep from feeling anything is to overeat. You've heard the phrase, "to stuff your face." Well, it could as easily be stated, "to stuff your feelings."

The surest road for getting through *anything* without eating over it is to get through *this* thing without eating over it. In other words, sit with your feelings. The feelings may have to do with a major life upheaval. Sit with them. More likely, the feelings you'd prefer to eat into oblivion result from everyday annoyances, nuisance situations, solvable problems that will work out whether you choose solution A or solution B. Whether you're meeting tragedy or trivia, you can sit with your feelings without food in your mouth. Each time you do this, the intensity of your desire to abuse food will mitigate and you will, perhaps without even knowing it, be inviting precious serenity into your world.

What it means to sit with your feelings is simply that, to *be* with them, to feel them, to come to know that they're not demonic forces but rather healers in their own right. Grief is a perfect example. Feeling grief, although certainly not enjoyable, is our part in the necessary process of recovering from a loss. Episodes of grief are precisely timed as if the body and mind share a well-set clock. You cannot grieve too much at once. There is some grieving now, later some more. Eventually, when the process has been allowed to complete itself, there is no more need for it.

Other emotions operate similarly. Anger fades. So does elation. They come to pass, not to stay. Every emotion has a purpose and a duration. To get in touch with these, understand them, act on them when appropriate and then let them go, it is necessary to be present to them. You can't do that while eating a hero sandwich, opening your mail, and watching the evening news. You do it by releasing the need for *doing* altogether and allowing yourself to simply *be*.

In our society-wide hastiness, it's easy to misinterpret feelings. What felt like hunger may be anger, shame, or fear. These feelings can manifest as a cold, empty sensation in the pit of your stomach. It's no wonder they are confused with the need for food. Lots of feelings can similarly be lost in translation. What seems like anger toward one person, for instance, may turn out to be anger toward someone else, or toward ourselves. What came to us as tension or anxiety could be the need to cry or talk or get a hug. In sitting with our feelings, we pay attention to them, the way a wise parent knows to pay attention to an unruly child, to learn what's behind the behavior.

Ideally, giving this sort of attention to feelings means taking some time to sit quietly and purposefully with whatever is going on inside you. This is a skill that will take some practice. You begin by not eating for the time being and choosing to do something with less potential for feelings-avoidance. Talking with an understanding person can be a godsend, as can writing in a journal, taking a walk, working in your garden, or availing yourself of a massage or some other sort of calming bodywork.

Eventually, you'll be able to sit—on a borrowed footstool maybe—with whatever is happening in and around you, and you won't be afraid. As you open yourself to what you feel, you'll find you become open to what you need. It may be a counselor, or a day off, or more fresh fruits and vegetables in your diet. You'll become aware of these things. What's more, you'll see that you *get* what you need.

I can remember when the prospect of voluntarily feeling what I was feeling without deadening it with food seemed about as likely as paying off the national debt from my Christmas savings. With enough reassurance from people who had done it, though, and with bits of practice whenever I could get it, I came to welcome opportunities to be present to my own interior life. It isn't always easy, but when you know that the only dependable way out of uncomfortable feelings is through them, the process becomes far less difficult to embrace. Fears decrease and boredom disappears. Problems cease being crosses to bear and become bridges to cross. And you'll come to expect something wonderful on the other side.

Peace with the Past

Two Buddhist monks were traveling on foot from their monastery to another in a neighboring town. To keep their vow of silence between sunrise and sunset, they walked wordlessly, reverently. After a few hours, they came to a flooded crossing. A finely dressed young woman was attempting to get to the other side, but there seemed no way for her to do this without soiling her garments from the water and mud. Seeing her plight, one of the monks approached her and, lifting her carefully, carried her across the rivulet. He then continued his journey. When darkness fell, the second monk admonished him, "I am shocked that, given our vows of purity, you blatantly touched a woman today!" "It is true," the first replied, "that I carried her in my arms over the water. But you, my brother, have carried her in your mind all day."[6]

6. This is the story as it was told to me by a friend several years ago. I later found another version of this story ("Muddy Road," p. 18), plus 100 other delightful ones, in *Zen Flesh, Zen Bones* compiled by Paul Reps (New York: Anchor Books, 1989).

We've already talked about living in the present. We don't take the first bite of a binge *today*. We sit with our feelings in *this* situation. To place ourselves firmly in the present, however, requires that we be at peace with the past. We cannot move gracefully through a current experience while lugging burdens of judgment, disappointment, guilt, and resentment that would, if examined, prove to be a burden of antiques. Like the accusing monk in the story, though, we can carry these burdens all day, and sometimes all our lives.

To deal sanely and compassionately with the past and with all the people in our lives, half of the Anonymous programs' Twelve Steps are devoted to personal inventory and personal peacemaking. Reread Steps 4 through 9 in Appendix D. You'll see that they begin with a thorough stocktaking (making a "searching and fearless moral inventory") and sharing what was discovered with oneself, another person, and a Higher Power.

It's important not to confuse this kind of inventory with something else, or to skip over it because you have done something similar before. It is not, as a case in point, putting yourself down or blaming yourself. In fact, the tendency to do that may come out in an inventory as something you wish to be free of. The inventory is not confession in the way you may know that term because you won't be looking for rules you have broken. Instead you'll find the actions and inaction that you yourself are uncomfortable with, that you wish you could change, that have or could lead you to unnecessary food.

The inventory is also not a digging for deeply buried psychological paraphernalia as you might with a professional in psychotherapy. Surely insights will present themselves that will be enlightening, but you needn't worry about uncovering information that is too much to handle. You will be taking a straightforward inventory of your character the way a shopkeeper inventories goods in a store. "A business which takes no regular inventory usually goes broke. Taking a commercial inventory is a fact-finding and a fact-facing process. It is an effort to discover the truth about the stock-in-trade. One object is to disclose damaged or unsalable goods, to get rid of them promptly and without regret. . . . We did the same thing with our lives."[7]

The most important aspect of an inventory is to do it. It is a neces-

7. *Alcoholics Anonymous,* p. 64.

sary part of your experiment in giving your poor, weary willpower a rest, in using Love's power from here on. There are many ways to take personal inventory, but the clear and basic procedure suggested in *Alcoholics Anonymous* is time-tested for success.[8] The recommendation there is for a three-part inventory covering resentments, fear, and sexuality.

The resentment list has three columns—one for the person or institution resented, a second for what he, she, or it did to cause the resentment, and a third for what that affects in you. As an example, you might write that you resent (first column) your sister, because (second column) she says you ought to lose weight, which affects (third column) your self-esteem.

The resentment inventory is both healing and informative. In column two when you are able to write about precisely what your resentments are, you're also recognizing feelings you may have denied for a long time. This is certainly healthy, but in itself it's not enough. To be free of a resentment, it is necessary to see what's going on in *you*—voila! column three. *Alcoholics Anonymous* cites self-esteem, pride, sexual relations, and finances as areas in our lives most likely to come up here, with fear underlying many of the difficulties with these. As you notice what comes out over and over in the third column, you'll be getting to know yourself much better.

The second part of the inventory is a list of fears. What are you afraid of? A sample fear list might look something like this:

· Losing my job
· Getting cancer
· Being fat forever
· Being hungry
· Flying
· Getting old

Whatever your fear, write it down. Keep writing as long as things occur to you. Nothing is too petty. If it comes to mind, it's in your heart, so put it on your inventory.

8. Detailed instructions for taking personal inventory may be found in *Alcoholics Anonymous*, pp. 64–71.

Our fears are also telling. The sample list shows insecurities around issues of health, safety, and finances. Some people have deeply embedded fears which can require special work, at times in a therapeutic setting, but many fear patterns can be traded for a faith response as soon as we decide to do so. Looking at the fears straight on is the first action necessary for making that switch.

The final part of the inventory concerns sexuality. Look at your past and present relationships and write about them. *Alcoholics Anonymous* suggests that you answer the following questions:

> Where had we been selfish, dishonest, or inconsiderate? Whom had we hurt? Did we unjustifiably arouse jealousy, suspicion, or bitterness? Where were we at fault, what should we have done instead? . . . . We subjected each relation to this test—was it selfish or not?[9]

You may find it helpful to add to these such additional queries as:

· Where have I allowed myself to be hurt?

· Have I settled for sex when I was looking for love?

· Do I accept myself as a sexual being?

· Is there balance in my sexuality—can I both respect and enjoy it?

Your answers are to provide insights into who you are, *not* provoke guilt feelings. An inventory is not an Inquisition!

If you do all three parts and you still feel that there's something missing, write whatever else comes to mind. And get a complete picture by topping off your inventory with a list of the things you admire and appreciate about yourself. False modesty is no good here. There are many splendid things about you. Write at least ten—better still, fifty. (And yes, it's okay for you to write that being a good cook is one of them.)

Then share the whole thing with another person. If you're in a Twelve Step group you can do this with someone who's done it already. Otherwise choose someone you trust to unjudgmentally accept you just as you are. Revealing the nooks and crannies of your soul to someone else, ideally someone who has seen and revealed nooks and

---

9. *Alcoholics Anonymous*, p. 69.

crannies of his/her own, brings a tremendous sense of peace. Some people feel that they're truly a part of life for the first time after sharing with another person, as well as with themselves and with the God of their understanding, exactly who they are.

We continue with the Twelve Steps' suggestions for cleaning up the past. Step 6 discusses our readiness to be without the character defects found in the inventory. It's amazing that we may actually want to hang on to shortcomings that have caused us pain and lured us to the kitchen. The fact is, we do often cling to them, just as we've clung to abusing food. There was a time we needed that food because we didn't have anything better. Now we do.

Similarly, we no longer need many of the defects of character that we had thought were necessary to make it in the world. When our lives are based on spiritual principles, we can prosper without dishonesty or manipulation because we are able to accept success as Love reaching out to us. We can meet our needs without interfering with others meeting their needs because we will realize that there is enough fulfillment to go around. And we can feel satisfied with the food we need to be healthy and full of energy without looking to extra or inferior food that promises satisfaction but only bogs us down.

When we ask that the troublesome parts of our personalities be taken away, we find that most are not so much removed as redeemed. A pushy personality becomes an outgoing, assertive one. Hypersensitivity is turned to sensitivity to the plight of other people, other creatures, and perhaps a heightened appreciation for art or nature. Low self-esteem is transformed into a humble self-acceptance and self-appreciation.

That word "humble" can have a red flag attached, and since Step 7 is worded "Humbly asked [God] to remove our shortcomings," this word deserves some attention. We confuse it with humiliation, which we as food addicts have so often suffered, instead of humility which most people, fat or thin, addicted or not, could handle a hearty helping of. Humility implies being who we are, not something other than that. And since we are already quite magnificent in our very humanness, why would anyone want to be more? Perhaps it's because we've often believed ourselves to be much less.

I like the status of humility conferred on Wilbur the pig in the children's book *Charlotte's Web*.[10] In it, Wilbur is spared from slaughter because his buddy, a literate spider named Charlotte, writes about him, by seemingly miraculous means, in her web. First come the accolades: Wilbur is "Some Pig," then he is "Terrific" and "Radiant." Charlotte's last weaving for her porcine companion is that he is "Humble." That may have been the highest tribute of all.

Making Peace

Steps 8 and 9 on the Twelve Step path discuss making peace with other people, or with ourselves regarding them. By going back to the inventory, you will see names of people you have hurt or with whom you have some discord. Without assigning the role of villain to you or them, you will see that these are people with whom there is outstanding acrimony that keeps you from balancing your life—the way checks too long outstanding can keep you from balancing your account. Step 8 involves listing those people and Step 9 involves making amends to those you've harmed if that's possible, " . . . except when to do so would injure them or others."

It may be my imagination, but I thought I just heard you say, "Huh-uh, not this one." There are plenty of reasons for wanting to bypass this Step. You could say:

- More people have harmed me than I ever harmed.
- He deserved what he got for what he did. (She did, too.)
- That creep is out of my life and I like it that way.
- I don't want to dredge up old dirt.
- This has nothing to do with how I eat.

I understand all these objections and each may have validity with the exception of the last. As human beings, human relationships motivate us more than any other factor beyond survival itself. We can deny their importance, but they are important nonetheless. *Relations with other people have a great deal to do with what, when, how, and why a person with a food problem eats.*

10. E. B. White, *Charlotte's Web* (New York: Harper & Row, 1952).

Be clear on what making amends entails. It is not groveling before another person, seeking his or her forgiveness, or reestablishing a partnership or friendship that has run its course. It is instead to *amend* the current, unsatisfactory situation. I think of person-to-person amends as something like amendments to the Constitution. The people who drafted the original document didn't look at it afterwards and say, "Oh, we left out freedom of speech and freedom of the press. Too bad." No, they *amended* what they had done with the Bill of Rights. That is what we need to do in our dealings with other people. We can amend (change, add to) our attitude or behavior toward them to make the relationship better.

Sometimes the best relationship is no relationship. That's fine. Your willingness to make each one the best that it can be is the goal. In some cases, amends can mean a simple apology. In others it can mean paying a monetary debt or making good on a promise. It can also mean putting your own name on top of your list and becoming fast friends with yourself. As you treat each situation in turn, you will find those "outstanding checks" coming in, and you'll be able to go to a new bank with evening hours and free checking. In other words, your life will be richer so your food won't have to be. Your life will be simpler so your food can be, too.

Expanding Your Comfort Zone

There once lived a widow woman who was always happy. She was at home in the parlors of the wealthy and titled who sought her counsel, and in the hovels of beggars to whom she brought cheer as well as bread and firewood. She delighted in the laughter of children and the ramblings of the elderly, in autumn leaves and spring flowers, in praying and in dancing.

In her town there lived a sorcerer. He was not an evil man, but he was selfish and used to getting his own way. He asked the widow woman for her daughter's hand in marriage. Now, she remembered something of marital bliss and not wanting her daughter to wed an old man, refused him. The sorcerer was angry and sought retribution.

First he brought fevered sickness upon the woman, but she still had the joy of her daughter's sweet voice and her many friends to nurse her back to health. Next the sorcerer condemned her to poverty. She and her daughter learned to forage for herbs and wild berries. On this frugal fare, the woman's face lost most of its lines and an annoying bit of rheumatism left her.

Further angered by the thwarting of his revenge, the sorcerer thought long on the perfect spell. "This one she will not overcome!" he vowed. Under the final curse, the woman was to have no peace, whatever the circumstances. She felt unfit to converse with the rich but too well-bred to associate with the poor, so she was lonely. Rain was too cold for her and sun too hot so she stayed indoors. Work seemed drudgery and play foolishness, so there was nothing to fill her hours. The woman was happy no longer.

She begged mercy of the sorcerer. "You have taken from me my most precious gift, the ability to be happy in any company and in any occupation. This was the greatest bequest I had to leave my daughter. Without it, I see no other way than to take her life and my own." The sorcerer's heart was moved to pity. "Woman, I see that what I seek is not your daughter's hand but her mother's secret." He lifted the curse and learned from the woman how to find contentment in every circumstance. And if you go to that town today, some will tell you that there is more to the story—that indeed the woman and the sorcerer were joined in marriage and lived many happy years together.

The woman in this little tale had a wide comfort zone. She found acceptance from everyone because she offered it to everyone, and she found joy in myriad activities because she looked for it in all of them. My friend Rita is like that. She loves opera, but she listens to country music on car trips so she can feel like a trucker. She knows about a million subjects, is convinced that she has never met an uninteresting person, and treats the world as if it were an amusement park to which she has a season pass. Rita has taught me a lot about comfort zones.

We all have one, that place or set of circumstances in which we feel safe, comfortable, unthreatened. We stray from its center in situations that are unfamiliar, or with which we have negative past associations. In these cases we tend to feel out of place; we may be uncomfortable with not knowing what to do or what's expected of us. It's only natural to feel more at ease in a friendly, familiar environment with people we know well, than in a strange place with strangers. Nevertheless, when we're grounded in the Love-powered life, when we start each day from Point Zero, *we carry an expandable comfort zone with us.*

When you bring these principles to life by living them, you will find that your serenity will no longer need to come from personal charm, although you may be charming, or from knowing the social graces, although you may be graced with every one of them, but from your Higher Power. You will be able to talk with your boss or a subordinate,

the President or some freckled friend of your ten-year-old and be genuinely interested in that person and genuinely secure in yourself.
You'll be looking across at people instead of up or down at any of
them.

The fine line between a frightening situation and an exciting one
will blur and your increasingly positive outlook will choose excitement over anxiety every time. Beyond this, however, you'll find that
your need for excitement will decrease and your preference for serenity will grow. Because you'll become proficient at getting what you
need, more and more serenity will become available to you.

Start where you are right now. Perhaps your comfort zone seems
small. You may think almost no place on earth is truly safe unless
you're armored with food or protective layers of fat. Don't despair if
you feel you're starting from the bottom. Start. Create your own safe,
nurturing, food-free, guilt-free comfort zone. At first, this may be a
private spot just for you. Then you can gradually expand it to include
one other person whom you trust, then others.

Your comfort zone may well be much broader than this at the outset, places or activities may still seem unsafe: supermarkets, interper-
sonal confrontations, speaking for groups. Allow your comfort zone
to grow. If you need to buy groceries, talk with a coworker about a
potentially volatile topic, or give a twenty-minute talk, use the same
techniques you did for sitting with your feelings, this time accepting
outer situations the way you then accepted inner ones. In this case,
instead of quietly being with your feelings, you can act in any given
instance—with your feelings or even in spite of them.

As you incorporate honesty, honest eating, facing feelings, and
letting go of the past into the framework of your life, *your comfort
zone will expand automatically.* You will find yourself in possession
of a degree of poise that may surprise you. You might attribute it
to a new haircut or to taking vitamins or losing ten pounds, and if
that helps—well, here's to haircuts. But as you encourage the flow-
ering of your spiritual self, you will come to see that *that* is the key
to your becoming more and more relaxed with whatever the day
presents.

No one has nonstop equanimity, but yours can increase exponen-
tially as you come to accept yourself more and more. As you do that,

you will also come to accept what is going on around you for precisely what it is at the moment, even those things that need to be changed. The more you are able to accept the way things are, the larger your comfort zone will become. This in no way means tolerating abuse or settling for less than you need. On the contrary, it means finding a centered spot in the midst of any circumstances. From that zone of comfort, from Point Zero, you can enjoy the positive and deal wisely and rationally with any negative elements that present themselves.

When my daughter was in kindergarten, I commented to her that a certain minor difficulty was really a blessing. "Disguised or the other kind?" she wanted to know. There is a place where the disguised ones are as valuable as the others, and blessings of every sort abound. That place is Point Zero. You may be there now as you read this book. If not, you're on your way.

◀ A MENTAL MAKEOVER ▶

Unproductive, negative thoughts can be turned into powerful, positive ones. Here are some examples of typical subzero self-talk and the respective Point Zero responses.

Subzero Thinking	Point Zero Responses
I don't measure up.	*I am adequate and more than adequate.*
I don't belong here.	*I am at home in my life and my world.*
Other people have their lives together.	*I refuse to compare how my life feels to how others' lives look.*
There's some secret to happiness but I don't have it.	*I discover something to feel happy about every day.*
If I could lose weight (or stop purging) my life would be in order.	*I live in an orderly way at my present weight.*
If my life were in order, I could lose weight (or stop purging).	*I eat in a loving way today regardless of outer circumstances.*

Subzero Thinking	Point Zero Responses
If I didn't manage everyone and everything, there would be chaos.	*I take care of my own responsibilities and leave the rest to God.*
If you knew the real me, you wouldn't like me.	*I am a likable person through and through.*
Things have been too good; I'm due for something awful.	*Things are good and I am grateful.*
Whatever it is is my fault (or your fault).	*My focus is on solving the problem, not assigning blame.*
I'm afraid of what will happen.	*I live in the safety of the present moment.*
I don't know what to do.	*I do the next thing indicated.*
I can't keep up the facade.	*I am who and what I am.*
If you would change, I could.	*I make the changes that are right for me regardless of anyone else's behavior.*
I know what to do, but I'm doing just the opposite.	*I know what to do and, alone or with help, I do it.*
I can't (try, start, risk, succeed) so I won't.	*I can (try, start, risk, succeed) and I'm doing it.*
I'm tired and I haven't done anything.	*I have plenty of energy to do what is mine to do.*
If I'm not perfect, I'm a failure.	*I am a perfect human being and perfect human beings have imperfections.*
Nobody else is like me.	*I am a member of the human family.*
I'm a special case.	*I'm a special person.*

◀ HONESTY EXERCISES ▶

- *Drive within the speed limit, even when you're sure you wouldn't get caught if you didn't.*
- *When you hear yourself putitng yourself down ("I'm a slob," "I can't do anything right"), change the tape. Blanket putdowns of yourself or others do not reflect the truth.*
- *When you're wrong, say so.*
- *If a certain food has always been a problem for you (i.e., "One bite is too many and a thousand aren't enough."), face it and leave that food alone.*
- *Abandon the coverup, for yourself or others. If you forgot to return a call, say "I forgot." If your child didn't do his or her homework, don't help out with a subterfuge.*
- *Share with someone else exactly what you're eating, or at least write down honestly what you're eating and share it with yourself.*
- *Shop for food honestly. Do you really need to serve the scout troop your favorite kind of cookie? Are you truly expecting someone who dearly loves chocolates to "just drop by?"*
- *Be completely honest about your life and your feelings with one or more people whom you trust.*
- *Eat the same way when you're alone as when you're with people and the same way with people as when you're alone.*
- *Be who you are wherever you are. If you have a chameleon suit, trade it in. Your beliefs, opinions, and preferences needn't be altered to fit one group or occasion and then another.*
- *When you find yourself exaggerating, bring the story down to size.*
- *Remember the important truth for food addicts: alone our prospects are grim, but there is a spiritual solution. Act on that truth.*

◀ FOOD FACTS FOR POINT ZERO ▶

Eating everything on your plate will not help a single starving child.[11] *Throwing away food you don't need is not terrible. If the food is good for your dog, feed it to the dog. If not, feed it to the earth via a compost pile.*

It is possible to get a fix from not eating just as it is from eating. *Do you get high from dieting or missing meals? Look at your behavior around food. Your goal is balance, to get food in its proper place in your life as a whole. That will mean diminishing its importance overall and not looking to food—either more than you need or less than you need—to feel better.*

You can prepare a meal without eating half of it in the process. *Follow an explicit recipe so you'll know the seasoning is right without tasting. If you do need to taste, do so at the end of the cooking process. A tiny taste will tell you all you need to know.*

If some food situations are particularly problematic, you can ask those around you for help. *As an example, if you've gotten into the habit of finishing off your children's leftovers while you clear the table, make getting the dishes to the sink or dishwasher and the scraps to the compost heap or garbage disposal their job, not yours. Eventually, that kind of temptation may not matter, but as long as it does, give yourself a break.*

There is no magical food that will make you lose weight or that will take away your appetite forever or anything like that. *Appreciate what is seemingly magical about food: that it can be transformed into what's needed to fuel one very important organism— you. If your relationship with food has been awful, approach it with an attitude that's more awe-filled.*

---

11. There actually are food choices you can make that can, in theory at least, help starving children. They're introduced in Chapter 6 and they don't require that you clean your plate!

Food is neutral, like water. *Water is a precious necessity, but it can also flood your basement, shrink your best pants, or even take your life. Similarly, food becomes a problem when it is misused or ill chosen. For this reason, your focus needs to be first on your life, then on your food.*

Wanting to lose weight is not the same thing as wanting to stop eating for a fix. *A heartfelt desire to live fix-free carries in itself tremendous spiritual power because it implies a willingness to live by the laws of nature and, if you will, of God. There's nothing wrong with desiring to lose weight simply to have a slimmer body, but spiritually it's about on par with wishing for a trip to Miami.*

You can say no to any food offered you by any person on this planet. *If that person is offended, there's a problem, but the problem isn't yours.*

—※—

FOUR

Looking In,

Reaching Out

I spent years of my life looking for a balance. I wanted the scale to balance on one number rather than another. But like watched pots that won't boil and counted chickens that refuse to hatch, that balance eluded me until another, more important balance was struck. That is the balance between my inner world and my outer one. In active food addiction one of those was invariably outweighing the other. Often I was caught up with work, other people, and frenzied activity, thereby avoiding who I really was. At other times, I stayed alone as much as possible, shielded with food, books, and television. The built-in isolation of eating for a fix kept me separated from both the richness of my interior world and of the world around me.

If you relate to that kind of separation, you can rest easy knowing that every day you live fix-free you will gently come more fully into the stream of life *in a balanced way*. Conversely, as you invite that fullness of life into your own experience, you will find that abstinence from unhealthful eating gradually becomes natural and effortless. *The task at hand has two parts: first, to look within through self-study, meditation, and prayer, then to reach out to others in friendship and service.*

Life is filled with such inner/outer dualities. Creativity, for example, needs an idea (internal) and expression (external). Each depends on the other. Artists don't lose their talents when they express them. On the contrary, every poem or painting refines, perfects, and intensifies the creative capacity of the person responsible for it. Along with your growing realization of your spiritual nature, your positive feelings and exuberance will actually increase as you share them with those around you and express them in all you do.

Understandably, a lot of people regard spirituality as optional at best because it appears to have to do only with intangibles. For addicts, however, those intangibles can get solid pretty fast. We *require* an active, sometimes intense, spiritual life in order to have a life worth living. **Our spirituality provides us with the wherewithal to deal with food, people, and problems just as surely as our work provides us with money for paying bills and going shopping.** Declining a spiritual life would do to our recovery what declining an income source would do to our buying power.

You may already acknowledge your spirituality. To bring it to bear on your food situation, you may need simply to expand that acknowledgment, to realize that food addiction affects the soul as well as the body, and that it is important enough to take to your God. Or perhaps you don't buy all this spirituality stuff. Self-examination may seem unnecessary and prayer ridiculous. Why pray if there's no one to hear? Why share and risk rejection? I think we look inside when we're tired of living with a stranger. We pray when we're tired of living alone, and we share because we're grateful that we're no longer tired.

You see, spirituality is like food and exercise. If you don't eat, you can survive on fat reserves, but not indefinitely. If you don't exercise, your muscle tone will last awhile, but not long. **Going within pro-**

vides you with spiritual food; giving to others is your spiritual aerobics. They work together.

◀ SPECIALIZING IN TRANSFORMATION ▶

This is still another difference between what we have done together so far and the other approaches that you've probably taken in an attempt to change the way you eat. Where diets and their kin focus on food, we've focussed on you and your relationship with the spiritual power within you that specializes in transformation.

That goes far beyond the mere restructuring of your body. When a physical change happens without the involvement of the rest of your being, it's doomed from the outset. It's no wonder that ninety percent of the people who lose twenty-five pounds or more regain it within only two years. They don't realize that the body is, ultimately, a reflection, a reflection of what is going on inside: emotionally, intellectually, and spiritually. A physical body of the proportions you fancy hasn't a chance of staying that way without the support of your heart, mind, and soul, without the support of your entire way of life.

Weight loss by itself is like winning the lottery. It's terrific, but many lottery winners, like weight losers, wake up at some point where they started, wondering what happened. What happened is that the recently rich aren't always able to develop the attitudes (emotion), knowledge (intellect), and/or consciousness (spirit) necessary to maintain prosperity: and the suddenly svelte usually lack the attitudes, knowledge, and/or consciousness to maintain slender bodies. (Attitude and consciousness are far more important than knowledge. With the right attitude and consciousness, you'll get the knowledge you need. You can, however, be a literal information bank on diet, nutrition, and the like, and still be caught in the morass of compulsive eating.)

Both the lottery winners and the weight losers had experienced a change in form—net worth or gross poundage—but *transformation* is more than that. Dr. Wayne Dyer, who does a lot of work with this idea, defines transformation as "going beyond form."[1] That's what

---

1. Dr. Wayne Dyer, *Transformation: You'll See It When You Believe It*, Tape #1, "Defining Transformation" (Chicago: Nightingale-Conant Corp.).

your Love-powered release of weight will be: a going beyond the form (this size or that, a larger waist measurement or a smaller one) to become the sort of person whose desires, preferences, and practices sustain a healthy, attractive body *as a matter of course.*

You have already realized that you can no more control your weight than you can control your grown children or the commodities market. What you are now doing instead is becoming someone for whom weight control is no longer an issue. *This proceeds from the inside out.* You've built a strong foundation while following the suggestions in the preceding chapters. Now you'll be looking at ways to guarantee daily renewal of the spiritual fitness necessary to keep food addiction at bay. That guarantee depends on keeping your life in ethical order, developing a viable relationship with the God of your understanding, and being of service to others as you put your entire life on a spiritual basis.

Remember that spiritual as we're using it could be defined as transformative or centered. It certainly *can* imply religious convictions, but for the purposes of leaving your addiction behind you, generic spirituality is quite adequate. Your personal spirituality can be nurtured on a continuing basis with the final three of the Twelve Steps. The first of these, Step 10, states: "Continued to take personal inventory and when we were wrong promptly admitted it."[2]

◀ ROUTINE MAINTENANCE ▶

Think of your character as a car. The moral inventory of Step 4 was a major tune-up: this ongoing, daily inventory is routine maintenance. When you take care of your car, you don't have to worry about driving it. When you take care of your life, you don't have to worry about living it.

Because we learn from mistakes, we're bound to make them as long as we're alive. We can't afford to deny them, rationalize them, or wallow in them. That's what ongoing inventory is about. *Alcoholics Anonymous* gives explicit instructions for how to go about this: "We continue to watch for selfishness, dishonesty, resentment, and fear. When these crop up, we ask God at once to remove them. We discuss

2. *Alcoholics Anonymous*, p. 59.

them with someone immediately and make amends quickly if we have harmed anyone. Then we resolutely turn our thoughts to some-one we can help."[3]

This is gratis guilt prevention. A mistake is like an accidental spill. Guilt is the stain that develops if it isn't cleaned up. Making instant amends most profoundly benefits *us*, but it also does wonders for our relations with others. We don't allow minor slights and misunder-standings to escalate into major ones. We don't allow the time to elapse in which our difficulties with another person could be taken to gossip court and tried by a jury of our peers.

Many people find it helpful to take a nightly mini-inventory in ad-dition to their daily lookout for selfishness, dishonesty, resentment, and fear. This inventory is a mental scan of the preceding waking hours to detect any unresolved disharmony or discomfort. Sometimes all you need to do here is forgive yourself and go to bed. Perhaps you'll want to offer a situation to your Higher Power or talk it over with someone. If something needs to be done about it tomorrow, make a note to that effect in your mind or in your journal, and tuck it away for the night.

◀ QUALITY TIME WITH GOD ▶

Before you go to sleep, spend a few quiet minutes with yourself and God. Have another quiet time in the morning before the demands of the day take all your attention. This is when you indulge yourself in the peacefulness of prayer and meditation. Certainly you can "pray without ceasing" in your thoughts and actions overall, and maintain the Buddhists' attitude of "mindfulness," a meditative appreciation of every moment as you go through your day. But setting aside some minutes specifically devoted to your inner life is necessary, too. You have quality time with your children. This is quality time with your God.

The Twelve Steps discuss this in Step 11 which says, "Sought through prayer and meditation to improve our conscious contact with God *as we understood Him,* praying only for knowledge of His will for

---

3. *Alcoholics Anonymous*, p. 84.

us and the power to carry that out."[4] For many people, this is an impelling invitation just as it's written, but if the word God doesn't give you feelings of warmth and peace, use another name or another image. Change "His will" to "Her will" if that, as the Quakers would say, "better speaks to your condition." A recovering alcoholic who writes anonymously as Rachel V. addresses this eloquently: "In [A.A.] meetings now I say that I'm promiscuous with God. I call on everyone: the Blessed Mother, the Lord Buddha, God the Father, Jesus Christ, Tara, the Holy Ghost, my Grandmother, Inanna, Kuan Yin, Isis, Ishtar, Kali, Sophia, the Shekina, anybody and everybody. I need all the help I can get. I'm sure that God understands. My life is evidence."[5]

Earmarking that kind of evidence in any of our lives is that balance between our inner and outer worlds. Prayer and meditation symbolize the balance exquisitely, because in them we reach out to a Higher Power by looking within to the place in ourselves where that Power resides. There is a myth in Hinduism that tells of the upset experienced by the gods after they created humans. They were afraid that this cocky species would discover divine truth and that people would then become gods themselves. To avoid being overtaken by upstarts, the gods tried to figure out where they might hide the truth out of humans' reach. If they hid it in the treetops, a person could climb there. If they hid it at the bottom of the sea, someone would dive down to discover it. The cleverest finally suggested, "Let us hide the truth deep inside every individual. That is one place they'll never look."

Well, sometimes we do. That's what prayer and meditation are about. Basically, prayer is talking to God and meditation is letting God answer. There is no single right way to do either one. If you follow a religious teaching, you have a wealth of information about prayer and meditation within your own religious tradition. As you explore it with renewed appreciation, you're apt to see a depth and beauty there that may have eluded you before. If you don't have such a tradition to draw on, you can still rest easy knowing that prayer comes naturally to hu-

4. *Alcoholics Anonymous*, p. 59.
5. Rachel V., *A Woman Like You: Life Stories of Women Recovering from Alcoholism and Addiction* (San Francisco, Harper & Row, 1985), pp. 210–11.

man beings as long as we don't get caught up in trivialities such as "thee" and "thou" and "ah-men" versus "a-men." If prayer is new to you, if you haven't tried it lately, or if you're feeling inhibited or skeptical about it, here are some suggestions.

How to Talk to God

Talk with your Higher Power the way you would talk with a friend. Don't bother thee-ing and thou-ing. Just talk — silently is fine. Share what's going on with you. If you feel foolish doing it, talk about that, too. *You can share anything*—even if it seems petty or you think God would disapprove. The loving God you're coming to know does not disapprove of you.

Read or commit to memory a couple of prayers that appeal to you. Think about the words and what they mean. ("A Prayer Primer" on page 69 lists some prayers you may want to try.)

In the morning, offer your day to God. Ask for help with your eating and for the decisions you will make that day. Ask to *remember* in the midst of all your activities that you're no longer by yourself.

Write to God. Put your thoughts, feelings, concerns, and delights down in a notebook or journal (see "To Keep a Journal" on page 73).

Start a prayer list or a prayer box. Put the names of people who are on your mind or situations beyond your control on a list in your notebook or in a small box or jar. Think of the names there when you have some quiet time.

Pray with your voice, your body, your creativity. Song, dance, and art can be powerful prayers.

Spend time in nature. Reverence is an effortless part of that.

Pray with someone else. This can be extremely uncomfortable at first, but if you persist with it, you'll find a special relationship developing not only between you and your Higher Power, but between you and the person with whom you're praying.

Explore affirmative prayer. Affirmative prayer is aligning our thoughts with God's through statements of divine truth. It's a way of opening ourselves to the blessings we've been ignoring but which are immediately available to us. Affirmations are positive statements like, "God loves me, so I love and care for my body."[6]

Most of us are used to praying *for* things, even bargaining—something like, "Get me out of this one and I'll do volunteer work twenty-two hours a week for the rest of my life." We have treated God like a celestial Santa Claus and when we don't get all the goodies on our list, we assume that prayer doesn't work or even that there is no God. It doesn't take much logic, however, to see that praying for things or for specific outcomes *couldn't* work in an orderly universe. I could pray for my side to win the war or the football game and you could pray for your side to win. Is God supposed to play favorites? Or someone could pray to lose weight while eating a banana split and planning to have another. That's asking for a circumvention of natural law and is about as absurd as praying, "You know, God, I'm really sick of all this gravitational pull. How about letting me float around fifty or sixty feet above ground for a while?"

Besides, praying for things and automatically getting them would mean avoiding the lessons we're here to learn. Learning from life is as inviolable a principle as the laws governing gravity or the metabolizing of that banana split. This may well be why Step 11 includes the phrase, "praying only for knowledge of His will for us and the power to carry that out." Now *that* can be horrifying. It's fine to let God have the cycles of nature and the orbiting of planets, but when it comes to *my* life, *my* relationships, and certainly the size of *my* jeans, I ought to know what's best! But you know what? I didn't know what was best all the time and I still don't.

Of course I can set goals, make choices, and steer my life in the direction that seems to be the proper one based on my intelligence, experience, and common sense. But intelligence, experience, and common sense aren't enough for a truly successful life. It also takes *uncommon sense*—intuition—and sometimes nothing short of Divine Providence. All prayers are answered, but sometimes when we pray

---

6. Affirmations can be useful mental exercises as well as a form of prayer. A good source for affirmations that deal with overeating is *Everything I Eat Makes Me Thin* by Richard Carlson, Ph.D., with Barbara Carlson (New York: Bantam Books, 1991), which says, "Instead of 'believing it when you see it,' start 'seeing it when you believe it.' This means that you must first decide that you are a thin, fit, and healthy person; then, and only then, will you allow yourself to become one" (p. 142).

for what we want the answer is no. When we pray instead for the will of the God that loves us in spite of anything, the answer is always yes, always right, and always best in the long run.

Years ago someone told me to stop praying for anything, even to stop overeating. "I only pray to be of service," she said. "Then I get everything else." I didn't trust that until I began to see it work in my own life. First, I stopped praying to lose weight. I prayed instead to live in keeping with the laws of life. The prayer was answered as the foods I selected changed and exercise that I actually enjoyed became a routine part of my life. Obesity cannot coexist with that lifestyle. I didn't have to pray to lose weight or work to lose weight. I prayed for God's will and, as my friend had also discovered, I got everything else.

Praying for God's will is not ignoring our problems and distresses. The Twelve Steps of Overeaters Anonymous explains, "Clearly, if we are to develop a vital relationship with a Higher Power, we will need to bring into our prayers all the things that concern us. We pray about these things, not so we can get our way, but so we can bring our will regarding them into alignment with God's will."[7] Lasting peace of mind and the ability to live fix-free depend upon that alignment.

Inner Listening

But how do we come to know what God's will for us is? Well, we just asked for it in prayer. Now it's time to wait for an answer. This brings us to meditation, the state of mental stillness in which the "still, small voice" may be heard. Sometimes called contemplation or contemplative prayer, meditation is found in all religious traditions and is also recommended by psychologists and health care providers as a means of stress reduction.

Simply stated, meditation is mental focusing. The object of that focus might be a word or syllable, an object such as a flower or candle flame, a phrase from a prayer or a scripture, or simply your own breath as you sit quietly observing your inhalations and exhalations, breathing in, breathing out, one breath at a time, no hurry, no worry, nothing to do but sit, watch, wait, breathe, listen. An easy but effective beginning meditation is to count your breaths. Count one on the in-

---

7. *The Twelve Steps of Overeaters Anonymous*, pp. 94–95. (See Appendix A.)

halation, and use a word such as Love, Peace, or Shalom to mark the exhalation. One, Peace; two, Peace; three, Peace; four, Peace, and so on until you reach ten. Then start again. (If you hit seventeen before you realize you've passed ten, gently bring yourself back to one. You're doing fine.)

When your mind wanders to what's on your desk at work, bring it back: one, Peace; two, Peace; three, Peace. . . . When your mind wanders to what to wear to the party this weekend, bring it back: four, Peace; five, Peace; six, Peace. . . . When your mind wanders to world affairs or your father's surgery or your teenager's SAT scores, bring it back: seven, Peace; eight, Peace; nine, Peace, ten, Peace. . . . Then start again: inhale one, exhale Peace; inhale two, exhale Peace. . . .

Do it for at least ten minutes in the morning. Morning and evening are better and twenty minutes in the morning and evening are best, but even a little meditation beats none at all. Your relief from addictive eating or obsessive weight control will come with living in the love you're offered by love's very Source. There is no substitute for connecting with that Source voluntarily, regularly, repeatedly. This may seem like a lot to do, but after you've made a place for prayer and meditation in your life as a whole, you'll wonder what you ever did without them. By reading about them and talking with people who already practice these spiritual disciplines, you'll devise your own routine for getting much needed inner nourishment.

Your way will fit your schedule and your temperament. I'll share with you what I do just by way of example. First, let me stress that I am not a marathon meditator. There are times I find it boring and would rather get on with the real highlights of life like bringing in the newspaper and feeding the cats. I do not hear voices, see visions, levitate or get any other noteworthy amusement from praying and meditating, nor would I want to. But I'm more peaceful than I used to be, and less afraid. My life works pretty well, and right now I'm thinking about writing this page instead of about something to eat. I believe that a great deal of the credit for this goes to the little bit of silence I take for myself virtually every day.

I start my day by recalling, even before I open my eyes, the realities that govern my life as a food addict: I cannot control food; that's the Higher Power's department; I renew my commitment to letting that Power deal with my life and my food for the upcoming twenty-four hours. Once I'm officially awake, I try to get to prayer and meditation right away. It doesn't always work out like this, but letting too many other things interfere can delete quiet time altogether.

Some people have a special chair or even a special room for meditation. I'm less formal. I usually sit up in bed Indian-style and start by writing in my journal. If there's something on my mind, it gets prayed out in pen and ink. If I'm feeling sorry for myself, I make a list of things I have to be grateful for. If the day ahead seems complicated, I write out my supposed obligations and see which of them really need to be done and which don't. In this way I clear my brain like orators clear their throats. Then I read something centering. I usually select something from one or two daily devotional books[8] but anything brief and inspirational will do. Then I close my eyes, check to see that I'm sitting in some semblance of erectness (I want to be alert for this), and allow my mind to mull over the words I've just read. When my thoughts go off in other directions, I bring them back to those words, to their ideas. Sometimes I need more structure and do the breath-counting meditation instead. In either case I finish with a prayer to do God's will that day. All of this takes about thirty minutes. Sometimes I cut it short. My best days are when I don't.

◀ SPAWNING MIRACLES ▶

At night I thank my Higher Power for the day. Some days have been filled with surprises and successes for which to be grateful. Other times I do well to say thanks that my food was okay and that the day is over. I often read a little nighttime thought from a book I like[9], but I don't have a bona fide bedtime meditation. At least I don't yet, but life is so much richer thanks to the modicum of inward turning I do already, surely any addition would be all to the good. Still, none of us needs to become a contemplative cleric to benefit from prayer and meditation. Concentrated quiet time at some point during the day

8. An excellent book of daily devotionals for people recovering from eating problems is *For Today* from Overeaters Anonymous (see Appendix A). *Daily Word* magazine (Unity School of Christianity, Unity Village, MO 64065) offers positive daily meditations with a nondenominational Christian orientation.
9. *Night Light, a Book of Nighttime Meditations*, by Amy E. Dunn, is excellent (from the Hazelden Meditation Series, see Appendix A).

and remembering the spiritual foundation of our lives and our recoveries the rest of the time are sufficient for spawning miracles.

Saying grace at meals is also especially appropriate for recovering food addicts. We can be thankful not only for having food to eat but for not abusing the food we have. If saying grace hasn't been a custom in your family, you may feel awkward about it at first, even about bringing it up with the people in your household. If that's the case, I suggest that you start to share a minute of silence before each meal. The people present can hold hands if they like. That minute may be used for a short prayer of gratitude, to remind yourself that the meal is in God's hands and you are, too, so you can eat without fear and without trying to meet emotional needs from what's on your plate. Those sixty seconds can also be a calming, centering time. Eating in that state of body and mind will make the food much more satisfying and it can even assist digestion.

Children are comfortable with graces and don't have nearly the inhibitions about them some adults do. My daughter has taught me some lovely ones. This one comes from schools that use the Waldorf system of education: "Earth who gives to us this food, Sun who makes it ripe and good, Dear Earth, Dear Sun, by you we live; our loving thanks to you we give." She adapted another from Robert Lewis Stevenson's *A Child's Garden of Verses*: "It is very nice to think the world is full of food and drink, and little children saying grace in every sort of holy place." (I'm also fond of the impromptu grace I overheard from a woman as she entered a buffet line: "Okay, God, You're on.")

It also makes sense to have an after-meals prayer. When we binged, meals never stopped. A prayer can give parameters we need. A Protestant friend of mine attended a Catholic Mass and took note of the priest's closing words, "The Mass has ended. Go in peace." She turned that into an after-eating prayer: "The meal has ended. I go in peace."

Indeed, to go in peace is how we can best leave a meal, a meditation, or any other activity. The peace that comes from giving our food problem to a Higher Power and from practicing prayer and meditation comes to life when we express it. Remember that balance of our inner and outer lives? This is it: turning what we receive from going within into sharing, caring, giving, and growing in our world, in our work, in our relationships.

Step 12 addresses this: "Having had a spiritual awakening as the result of these steps, we tried to carry this message to [others] and to practice these principles in all our affairs."[10] Only this Step includes the verb "to try." The others are quite clearly to be done, but because carrying the message implies a response from someone else, it can only be tried, attempted. What the other person does with it is up to that person.

If you've taken advantage of the tremendous help that's available by contacting other recovering food addicts, you know that people who are putting these principles to work for themselves have turned theory into fact in a most impressive way. Regarding some things, we're all Missourians. We addicts need to be *shown* that spirituality isn't just Pollyanna pleasantness but that it can actually bring people from obsession, obesity, and despair to lives that are in order, bodies that are healthy and comfortable, and outlooks that are hopeful with good reason to be so. You can in turn offer this to others.

You don't need to wait until you're thin (that will eventually happen) or until you're perfect (that will never happen) to be of service to someone else. When I first began to look for a spiritual solution to binge-eating, I was put in touch with a woman who proved to be very helpful. We had a wonderful long-distance conversation and just before our good-byes she said, "Now call someone and give them whatever you've gotten from this talk." "But I can't do that," I protested. "I just binged last night!" "There's someone out there who binged this morning," she replied. "You've got something they need."

I did what she told me. I called someone that I knew used food the way I did and let her know what I'd learned. Of course, I had to tell her that I was no expert and had only binged the night before. What I see now, though, is that no recovering addict is ever an expert. Any of us could choose to go back to old ways of thought and action and would be abusing food again in no time. Addicts who stay in recovery live in blessed moments, in the now, in a state of grace that keeps anxiety at bay. Because our new lives do not come from us as ego-entities, we can only share with others in the company of good old humility.

10. The Step as originally presented by Alcoholics Anonymous reads, "to carry this message to alcoholics . . ." (*Alcoholics Anonymous*, p. 60). Other groups which use the Twelve Steps change "alcoholics" to "overeaters," "addicts," etc.

Once you're thin, it is possible that you may want to forget where you came from. A long while back, after I lost weight through a commercial diet program, I got a job there. Everything went fine at first. But then I stopped relating to the people who came there for help. One day I unloaded to a coworker: "I am so sick of being around fat women!" It wasn't two weeks before I was back to binge-eating and a huge, rapid weight gain. At the time I hadn't a clue that I couldn't deal with those "fat women" because I was one of them. I had not accepted my addiction, my vulnerability or, to a great extent, my humanity. Going back to overeating was inevitable.

You can avoid such pitfalls by remembering Love as your power source. In a support group, you'll have ample opportunities to share, but life itself offers such chances, too. People will ask how you lost weight or they'll comment on how much happier or calmer you seem. When they do, tell them a little. If they're interested, they'll ask for more. The idea is to offer what you have without force-feeding anyone. It's possible for your enthusiasm to come across as fanatic zeal, leaving the impression that you've seen the light and are ready to outfit everybody else with the sunglasses they're sure to need shortly. It's important to tone that down. When you're established in recovery, you won't be out to make converts or reach a quota, but simply to be a resource about what made the difference for you.

One way to avoid being pushy is to speak with "I" messages instead of "you" messages. An "I" message is saying, "I found that I needed a spiritual solution for my food problem" rather than, "If you'd get some spirituality in your life, you could stop overeating." You've heard the old adage, "Your actions speak so loudly I can't hear the words you say." It's true. Our actions are chattering all the time, sometimes in shouts, sometimes in whispers, but they're always heard. When you have had a spiritual awakening, your life itself will carry the message—not just to other food addicts but to everyone you contact.

◄ HUNGRY FOR HARMONY ►

People are hungry for greater harmony, peace, and understanding in their lives. Without these, some overeat; some overdrink; some overworry. Others stay moderate in their habits but never achieve more than moderate happiness. For people like these, just being in the same room with you when you have achieved inner peace could change their day. Being your friend could change their destiny. That's because *disease* isn't the only thing that can be contagious. *Ease* can be contagious, too. In the same way that looking to others to be role models and confidantes is invaluable in your recovery, being those things to other people will give your recovery strength and longevity.

It is that strong, day-by-day recovery that makes it *possible* to "practice these principles in all our affairs." These principles will be obvious in your total way of living, and we'll explore this further in Chapter 9, "The Love-Powered Life." Right now, though, while we're thinking about reaching out to others, let's consider how to incorporate our new ideals into personal relationships. It begins with the inventory Steps and making amends. As your recovery progresses, you'll find yourself attracted to healthier relationships just as you'll be attracted to healthier foods.

As you continue with persistence and the willingness to let your Higher Power work *in every area of your life*, you'll find yourself living what at first seems to be a paradox. You will love people more but you'll be less attached. You'll be able to let go emotionally, freeing the people you care about to be themselves, their best selves. You'll stop trying to control other people, similar to the way you'll have stopped trying to control your food and your weight. You will accept people precisely as they are because you accept yourself precisely as you are.

There are plenty of good books available on improving relationships, and you may find them helpful for learning techniques of better communication and of relating more confidently to others. Strictly by virtue of what is taking place within you as you overcome your addiction, however, you can *expect* your dealings with those around you to improve. If they don't, you'll be equipped to take positive action. Unhealthy relationships that you may have tolerated before your Love-empowerment began will be like the clothes you wore then: they'll require some alterations.

Be patient with those who are watching you change. Another's transformation can be threatening. Those you love need to know that you're not abandoning them as you become more fully who you really are. On the other hand, never allow another's fear of your growth to impede it. Your primary obligation is to your own unfolding. When you are committed to that, your commitment to your family, friends, and colleagues will have the best possible foundation.

Looking within for guidance and reaching out to get and give more of the same will make you a better friend and a better partner—not just to other people in your life, but to yourself. You will treat others with fairness and respect and you will accept no less from them. *You'll be learning to love in the truest sense of the word because you'll be learning from Love itself.* This is part of how the process works, part of the way your thinking/feeling nature must work if you are to live addiction-free. If you came to this way of life only hoping to lose weight, this is one remarkable bonus.

- - - - - - - - - - - - - - -

A PRAYER PRIMER

I was once told that it's important to have prayers, poems, and uplifting quotations filed away in my memory bank because there would be times I'd be alone with only what was in my mind. If I'd stored away words of beauty and inspiration, they would be there for me. I have found that to be true. Some of those that serve me well I've included here. Feel free to choose from these (many of which will be familiar to you) or find your own. You never need to use prewritten prayers in order to talk with your Higher Power, but they do make good company.[11]

THE SERENITY PRAYER

God, grant me the serenity to accept the things I cannot change,
The courage to change the things I can,
And the wisdom to know the difference.

11. Since these are given in traditional form, the language is sometimes formal and the pronouns are often masculine. Change whatever you need to or skip an offending prayer altogether. The same applies to theological references that are not in keeping with your personal beliefs.

THE LORD'S PRAYER

Our Father who art in heaven, Hallowed be thy name. Thy kingdom
  come. Thy will be done in earth, as it is in heaven.
Give us this day our daily bread.
And forgive us our debts, as we forgive our debtors.
And lead us not into temptation, but deliver us from evil:
For thine is the kingdom, and the power, and the glory, for ever.

A SIKH DEVOTION (from the *Asi Ki War*)

Wonderful Thy word, wonderful Thy knowledge;
Wonderful Thy creatures, wonderful their species;
Wonderful their forms, wonderful their colors;
Wonderful the animals which wander naked;
Wonderful Thy wind; wonderful Thy water;
Wonderful Thy fire which sporteth wondrously;
Wonderful the earth, wonderful the sources of production;
Wonderful the pleasures to which mortals are attached;
Wonderful is meeting, wonderful parting from Thee;
Wonderful is hunger, wonderful repletion;
Wonderful Thy praises, wonderful Thy eulogies;
Wonderful the desert, wonderful the road;
Wonderful Thy nearness, wonderful Thy remoteness;
Wonderful to behold Thee present.
Beholding these wonderful things I remain wondering.

THE PRAYER FOR PROTECTION, by James Dillet Freeman[12]

The light of God surrounds me.
The love of God enfolds me.
The power of God protects me.
The presence of God watches over me.
Wherever I am, God is.

---

12. "The Prayer for Protection" was first published by Unity School of Christianity and is reprinted with permission.

A HINDU PRAYER

Lead me from the unreal to the Real.
Lead me from darkness to Light.
Lead me from death to the knowledge of Immortality.
May the entire world be happy.

A PRAYER OF ST. FRANCIS

Lord, make me an instrument of your peace.
Where there is hatred, let me bring love.
Where there is injury, let me bring pardon.
Where there is discord, let me bring harmony.
Where there is error, let me bring truth.
Where there is doubt, let me bring faith.
Where there is despair, let me bring hope.
Where there is darkness, let me bring light.
Where there is sadness, let me bring joy.
Lord, grant that I may seek not so much
To be comforted as to comfort,
To be understood as to understand,
To be loved as to love.
For it is in seeking that we find.
It is in forgiving that we are forgiven.
It is in dying to the things of self
That we are born to Eternal Life.

AN ANTHROPOSOPHICAL PRAYER, by Rudolph Steiner

May the events that seek me come unto me.
May I receive them through the
    Father's ground of peace on which we walk.
May the people who seek me come unto me.
May I receive them with an understanding heart through the
    Christ's stream of love in which we live.
May the spirits that seek me come unto me.
May I receive them with a clean soul through the
    Healing Spirit's light by which we see.

THE TWENTY-THIRD PSALM

The Lord is my shepherd; I shall not want.
He maketh me to lie down in green pastures; he leadeth me beside the
  still waters.
He restoreth my soul; he leadeth me in the paths of righteousness for
  his name's sake.
Yea, though I walk through the valley of the shadow of death,
I will fear no evil: for thou are with me; thy rod and thy staff they
  comfort me.
Thou preparest a table before me in the presence of mine enemies;
  thou annointest my head with oil; my cup runneth over.
Surely goodness and mercy shall follow me all the days of my life: and
  I will dwell in the house of the Lord for ever.

From "ON PRAYER," *The Prophet*, by Kahlil Gibran

"Our God, who art our winged self, it is thy will in us that willeth.
It is thy desire in us that desireth.
It is thy urge in us that would turn our nights, which are thine, into
  days which are thine also.
We cannot ask thee for aught, for thou knowest our needs before they
  are born in us:
Thou art our need; and in giving us more of thyself thou givest us all."

THE GREAT INVOCATION

From the point of Love within the Heart of God
    Let love stream forth into the hearts of men.
        May Christ return to Earth.
From the center where the Will of God is known
    Let purpose guide the little wills of men—
        The purpose which the Masters know and serve.
From the center which we call the race of men
    Let the Plan of Love and Light work out
        And may it seal the door where evil dwells.
Let Light and Love and Power restore the Plan on Earth.

NATIVE AMERICAN PRAYER

Now Talking God
With your feet I walk.
I walk with your limbs.
I carry forth your body.
For me your mind thinks;
Your voice speaks for me.
Beauty is before me
And beauty behind me;
Above and below me hovers the beautiful:
I am surrounded by it,
I am immersed in it.
In my youth I am aware of it
And in old age I shall walk quietly
The beautiful trail.

◀ TO KEEP A JOURNAL ▶

There are many ways to pray and meditate. You can be in your house or in a church, on the beach or on the bus. You can pray and meditate in the lotus position or in a chair, kneeling or walking. And you can communicate with yourself and your God with thoughts or words, or on a sheet of paper, or better yet on many sheets of paper in a daily journal.

A spiritual journal entails much more than keeping a diary or calendar, although it can incorporate those functions. The real purpose of a spiritual journal is to facilitate your inner growth. How it does this specifically depends upon you and what you want to achieve, but a journal can be used in any of the following ways:

1. Write in it first thing in the morning to become grounded in the day at hand. There's something about writing today's date that implies a commitment to the nonrefundable span of time you'll have to spend during this day.

2. Record your food, either as a flexible plan for the day ahead or, in the evening, as a record of the gift of sane eating you received.

3. Describe your feelings when you're feeling a lot of anything, even if you can't label the feelings right away.

4. Write about decisions you have to make. List the pros and cons of your choices. This will help to clear your thinking process.

5. Write down what you need to do for the day. If there are forty-four things to do in a twenty-four-hour day, laugh. Then make cuts.

6. Write out affirmations. It's fine to speak statements of universal truth but when you write them, especially if you do it several times a day for a month or so, they become your statements of personal truth.

7. Write letters to God (instant delivery, quicker than a fax).

8. Write down ideas that you see or hear and want to internalize. Whether the thought comes from great literature or a bumper sticker, put it in your journal and assume that it will find its way into your life as if by osmosis.

9. At night, empty your day into your journal. Make note of what you learned and what you're thankful for. If you do a personal inventory in the evening, this can go in your journal, too.

The mechanics of keeping a journal aren't really important. You can buy very attractive, clothbound books with blank pages and write in those, but if you have a practical nature like I do you'll prefer a spiral notebook that stays flat and provides you with lines to write on. Be sure to write with a pen that feels good in your hand and glides easily across the paper: You can't "go with the flow" when your ballpoint is sticking. And don't fret about spelling or punctuation: your English teacher retired.

Sometimes people are wary of keeping journals because of the personal nature of what might be written there. Fortunately, most of us either have lives that are much less interesting than we think or handwriting so poor the curious wouldn't bother to decipher it. Unless you have special circumstances, your journal is probably quite safe in a drawer in your desk or nightstand. If you write something you'd rather no one ever sees, tear out the page and destroy it. It's yours to do with as you like.

You can also choose to share the contents of your journal with another person. Sometimes our true thoughts and feelings come out much more lucidly when we're writing in a journal than when we're trying to speak extemporaneously. (A dear person once said to me, "You'd better write it down: I've known you to put your foot in your mouth, but almost never in your typewriter.")

You can save each journal you finish and go back to earlier ones as personalized reference books for your ongoing growth. Old journals can be solid evidence of how far you've come on days when you doubt your progress. They're also testimonials to everything you've come through with the help of your Higher Power. You will appreciate this resource when you are faced with difficulties that seem insurmountable. On the other hand, a Love-powered life is the life you live today. In this respect, an outdated journal is so much kindling.

If you can use a record of the past to enrich the present, keep your completed journals. Otherwise, clear away the space they take in your drawer and in your psyche. This is a new day. Write the date on top of the page. Claim it. It's yours.

- - - - - - - - - - - - - - - - -

◀ MORE REVOLUTIONARY CONCEPTS ▶

The revolutionary concepts introduced in Chapter 2 had to do with you as a person and your relationship with food. The following ideas are revolutionary as well, but they pertain to you as a friend and partner and to your relationships with the people in your life. Read them every day this month.

Recovery will touch every aspect of your life. You cannot change the way you relate to God, yourself, and food without also changing for the better the way you relate to other people.

·

If you have tried to control your food and your weight, you have probably tried to control people, too.

You have one life: your own. No one else's life belongs to you, not even your spouse's or your children's.

·

You may truly believe you know what other people should do, but that doesn't mean they'll do it or even that it's your job to tell them. Just share your own experience.

·

No one makes you feel one way or another. You can decide how you'll feel.

·

Pleasing other people is fine as long as it pleases you, too. That doesn't mean you should never be self-sacrificing: Just be sure you want to do something for someone else before you do it, so you don't end up resenting it.

·

You can listen compassionately to another person without feeling that you have to fix that person's life or situation.

·

There is no better way to make a positive connection with another person than by being exactly who you are. You are the best you on record, and your genuineness will be recognized by the genuine part of another person.

·

The way to avoid having misunderstandings in relationships is to have no relationships. Having challenges in a relationship does not prove you a failure; it proves that you and the other person involved are human.

·

Your opinions are as valid, your needs as important, and your life as valuable as anyone else's. (This is true now, regardless of anything you have done; anything that has been done to you; how much you weigh; or what anyone says or thinks of you.)

·

What other people think is not of your concern. As long as you're true to yourself, let others think what they like. (They will anyway.)

Not every relationship is meant to last forever, and even those that last change.

·

Having a relationship with food is much less difficult than having a relationship with a human being. However, the latter is more reward-ing and won't give you heartburn.

·

Addictive people can have more than one addiction. An addictive re-lationship—one that is damaging but seemingly impossible to change or end—can impede your recovery. If you suspect that you need professional help or group support in this area, get it.

- - - - - - - - - - - - - - - - -

❧ STRIKING THE BALANCE ☙

Keeping your recovery strong and viable will rest on two responsibil-ities: continued surrender of your eating problem to a Higher Power and maintaining the balance of a healthy spiritual life and a healthy life, spiritually lived. The following suggestions may help you come to this balance of "looking in, reaching out":

Make personal inventory an ongoing practice. *Be on the look-out for "selfishness, dishonesty, resentment, and fear." When you see these, be prepared to let your Higher Power take them, to discuss them with another person, make apologies or take other action if in-dicated, and set your mind on how you can help others.*[13]

Review your day before you go to sleep. *Is there something you want to talk about with God or another person? Is there something you would like to handle differently the next time it comes up? Is there some situation left from today that you want to be sure to take care of tomorrow? What progress have you seen in yourself today? What is there in your day that pleases you or that you can be proud of? Thank your Higher Power, and give yourself some credit, too. You're doing great.*

13. See *Alcoholics Anonymous*, p. 84.

Pray and meditate every day. It was suggested back in Chapter 2 that you take some quiet time for yourself each day. Prayer and meditation are simply a continuation and expansion of that. You can use your quiet time to read something soothing or inspiring, to write in your journal, to read or say any prayers that are meaningful to you, to talk with God about what's on your mind, or to tend to the specific devotions that may be part of your own religious faith. Do use some of this time for silent meditation, using the breath-counting technique or another method to still your mind and be open to your Higher Power.

Share what you have found with others. Sharing is offering, not forcing. As you recover, you will find ways to share nonintrusively and beneficially, particularly if you are part of a support group for recovering food addicts. Remember, too, that your life itself carries the message to other food addicts and to everyone around you.

Remember your new way of life in all your activities and relationships. As someone relying on spiritual truths to recover from food obsession, you will be living a spiritual life. This doesn't imply prudish piety. It does imply putting all your actions and your dealings with people on a spiritual basis. As you live this new way and make contact with your Higher Power in prayer and meditation, much of this will come to you intuitively. You will look for something of God in everyone around you. You will allow other people to be who they are. You will be able to accept others as they are and, perhaps especially, yourself as you are.

—✻—

FIVE

The Gift

of Choice

You have embarked on an inner journey. Its destination, spiritual awakening, is not like a port or a station. You won't arrive, unpack your bags, and have done with it. It is instead the opening of a door to a new way of life, one lived on a daily basis, renewable every morning. And every morning a spiritual gift will be waiting for you, just as surely as if it were a package in wrapping paper with your name on the tag. That is the gift of choice.

There is no choice in eating for a fix. We did it when we thought we wanted to and when we knew we didn't, yet the idea of refraining from it was paralyzing because we thought it meant our choice would be taken away. In truth, however, it is only when we're relieved from having to overeat or undereat, reward ourselves with food or punish ourselves with deprivation, that we really have a choice at all. Only then can we make choices about our lives—to treat ourselves well, for example—*and* about our food.

As a recovering food addict, you will need to learn how to use the gift of choice the same way you have learned to use tangible gifts, from your first bike to your personal computer. In the throes of the addiction, many choices were limited. You wore an outfit because it was the one that fit. Perhaps you took a certain job because you didn't feel good enough about yourself to apply for the other one, the one you really wanted. And if you're like me, you certainly ate some particular food or other not because you really wanted it or even because it tasted all that great, but because it was around, or because it was the one that offered the kick or the sedation needed at the time.

In recovery, choices abound. With a reprieve[1] from food obsession and a commitment to Love-powered rather than ego-powered living, you will be able to choose to

- Believe you're okay because "God doesn't make junk"
- Accept life instead of fighting it
- Go with Love instead of fear
- Feel good physically and emotionally
- Forgive yourself and others
- Reach out to people
- Find humor in almost every situation
- Take good care of yourself
- Be grateful
- Express your feelings
- Experience compassion
- Have fun
- Welcome supportive friends into your world
- Give to life and enjoy the rewards of giving
- Ease up on yourself
- Take risks
- Look on the bright side
- Rejoice in others' good fortune as well as your own
- Delight in the little things

---

1. *Alcoholics Anonymous*, p. 85: "We are not cured of alcoholism. What we really have is a daily reprieve contingent on the maintenance of our spiritual condition. Every day is a day when we must carry the vision of God's will into all our activities."

- Feel attractive
- Smile
- Unleash your creativity
- Learn from difficulties
- See the beauty around you
- Put more beauty around you

- Be honest
- Look forward to every day
- Grow
- Love
- Be happy

Can you see that all these things are choices? Does it make sense to you that we can choose, for example, to be happy, or does it seem that happiness has to happen *to* us, that it is the *result* of a hefty raise, a smart purchase, a fresh compliment? Of course these things give us a boost. It's wonderful when they happen. That boost, however, is not happiness. Happiness is far less flighty. It comes from within and depends on little else. It is a choice.

In Dr. Wayne Dyer's charming fantasy-with-a-message, *Gifts from Eykis,*[2] an earthling travels to another planet and finds that everything there is identical to earth except people's psyches. There anxiety is an entity that actually *attacks*, and news broadcasts warn of airborne anxiety levels the way ours report pollen counts for those suffering from hay fever. But anxiety doesn't attack on our planet. Neither does unhappiness. Oh, there is no lack of challenges, or of dilemmas, problems, and losses, even severe ones. That frustration, anger, and grief will be experienced regarding these is natural, but your underlying sense of well-being (happiness) will still be with you if you choose to have it.

There certainly may be times when you'll choose to feel unhappy. That's all right. You might want to give yourself an unhappiness allotment of an hour or two and then get on with whatever it takes to put you back in touch with the reality that you can indeed choose to be happy. "Whatever it takes" will probably be one of the same methods you're already using to postpone inappropriate eating: talking with another person, getting a change of scenery, or having a quiet time for prayer, journal writing, or meditation. Do what you need to. It isn't always easy to remember that you're choosing your own feelings—

2. Dr. Wayne Dyer, *Gifts from Eykis* (New York: Simon & Schuster, 1983).

sometimes it can seem as if anxiety is attacking in a way that's down-right extraterrestrial!

Even so, you can go on the *premise* that all these choices are yours and you'll see that the premise is correct. The ability to make choices is a gift from Love to you, and you're at liberty to do just that. There are two choices, though, that recovering food addicts need to make each day. The first is *to choose to remember that our lives have been turned over to the care of a Higher Power*. If you're working the Twelve Steps, you made your original decision to let that Power take care of your will and your life back at Step 3. That step could be likened to deciding to take a job. Choosing *each day* to remember the decision to keep things in God's hands is like showing up for work at nine o'clock prepared to do the best you can.

When you operate from the proposition that your Higher Power (God, Love, Spirit, Higher Self) is handling the outcome of situations, you can do what you do best: take care of what is in front of you. Don't believe for a minute that this means resigning yourself to dullness, drudgery, and an uneventful life. When you team up with the power of Love, what will be in front of you to do will oftentimes surpass your wildest dreams. Of course there will be *some* dullness, drudgery, and uneventfulness. Everybody has that. But Love provides bright spray paint for even the grayest of times and chores.

The second important daily choice for continued recovery is *to choose to refrain from eating for a fix*. You actively implement this choice every time you use the postponement techniques, and every time you elect to sit with your feelings without something to eat, drink, or chew for the time being. Therefore, you are already aware that to choose to refrain from eating for a fix bears little resemblance to going on a willpower diet. Diets can, in fact, impede progress because they give the illusion that we can control our eating which, for any true food addict, is a dangerous fallacy. What is required in terms of food choices is a new way of eating that arises from the new way of thinking provided by a spiritual approach to life.

As your recovery proceeds and you reconfirm each day your commitment to your Higher Power, you will experience with growing frequency that choosing not to eat for a fix won't even seem like making a choice. It will be a non–issue, in the same category as having to choose whether to buy a jet this month or a small island in the Caribbean. That degree of freedom is incredible for those of us who have known not being able to get through just one hour without obsessing over food. Nevertheless, eating for a fix can be virtually *guaranteed* any food addict who goes back to former patterns of thought and action. Therefore, whenever you keep harmful or unnecessary food out of your mouth—even if this requires no conscious effort because you simply don't want the food—you have already made the choice to refrain from eating for a fix. You are unconsciously acting on that, and your appetite itself has, in fact, responded to the choice you have made.

I call these times "state of grace days" because we don't have to earn them. We only have to accept them. Expect to enjoy ever greater numbers of these as time goes by. On some days, though—and in the beginning, it may be all days—you'll still want to eat the way you always have. This is not terrible and it does not mean that you are a failure! It most likely means one of two things. The first possibility is that there is something missing in your spiritual life. Use the opportunity to look at your recovery practices. Do you recognize that your own power is useless when it comes to food? Are you looking to your Higher Power for help? Are you willing to postpone the fix and to sit with your feelings? Do you need to let go of some shame or guilt or resentment that hasn't been dealt with? Would it help to talk things over with someone? Do you owe amends? Have you been taking time for prayer and meditation? Are you sharing with others? Are you using spiritual principles in all aspects of your life, those that have to do with your eating and those that don't? Sometimes taking *a single action* to deepen your spiritual life can rid you of the most stubborn food craving. If you can't pinpoint exactly what's amiss, just do *something*. Take half an hour for journal writing and meditating, or call someone whom you know is having a difficult time and offer that person a patient ear.

A second reason you may be experiencing the desire to overeat could be physical. Perhaps you recently ate a particular food that, for you, incited an obsessive pattern (see the section in Chapter 6 on binge foods) or there may be a lack of balance in your physical/emotional self. The Anonymous programs use the acronym HALT to remind their members not to get too *hungry*, too *angry*, too *lonely*, or too *tired*. When you want to extend a meal beyond reasonable parameters or eat what you know is extra, unnecessary food between meals, examine your life in terms of HALT. You may have two or three of the danger signals operating without realizing it. Take care of them. This is another reason to stay away from diets. On most of them, you're hungry from lack of food; angry about being on a diet; lonely because so much socializing takes place around food; and tired from lack of nutrients or from trying to restrain yourself.

On those hungry days, you'll need to make the conscious choice not to eat for a fix—and you may need to do it more than once. The difference between choosing to abstain from damaging eating and using willpower to stick to a diet is surrender versus combat. When you surrender the inclination, desire, or compulsion to misuse food to the Power of Love, the struggle is over.

◄ A WILLOW'S FLEXIBILITY ►

And you can surrender perfectionism at the same time. **When you are no longer eating for a fix, you will still sometimes eat more than you need. You might make a food choice that you wish afterwards had been different. When these things happen, you will not have "broken your diet" because there is nothing to break.** You will have a willow's flexibility to withstand storms that would demolish an oak. Without having to reach some nebulous state of perfection, either in your life or at your meals, you will be living out your choice to be fix-free each day.

Another choice that will be yours in recovery is that of choosing what you will eat. You don't simply stop and stay stopped as you might with another addiction. You need to stop *abusing* food but still decide what to fix or what to order for breakfast, lunch, and dinner. Knowing what to eat and how much can be scary. After all, food seems to have been the cause of so much misery. How do you know you can trust it, or that you can trust yourself to make decisions about it?

You may remember times that you fasted or went on liquid diets and felt a peacefulness that eluded you when you had to return to eating solid food. Part of the appeal of such programs is that with them you don't need to have anything to do with food—out of sight, out of mind, so to speak. But just as you can't learn to swim on dry land, you can't learn to eat in a loving way, or even come to know that it's possible, until you try it.

The inner change you're offered will render you capable of dealing with life as it is. Part of this life is to eat, for human beings and every other animal on the planet. Although every addict who expects to get well must respect the severity of addiction, fear doesn't heal anybody. Love does the healing, and love and fear cannot work in the same space. If you are afraid of food, put that on the fear list in your personal inventory and ask your Higher Power to take the fear away. St. John once said, "Perfect love casts out fear," and this still applies. You can *expect* to develop a new, respectful but fearless attitude toward food.

If you started turning to food when you were a child, you evidently needed that to shield you from things you feared, or that you didn't understand or could not handle. Many people with eating disorders were physically, mentally, or sexually abused as children,[3] but even in happy homes, some needs go unmet. Then, the food was a friend, a helper, a protector. It can't help you anymore and you don't need its brand of protection, but it can become a friend in a sane, mature manner, the way you may now admire and enjoy a sibling that you envied and resented as a child. Your attitude has changed. Your attitude toward food can change as well.

As your attitude changes, you will make food choices from a different vantage point. When, for example, you were eating for emotional solace, you may have gravitated toward sweet, creamy foods that were usually high in fat and nutritionally marginal. With a different motivation for eating—the desire to nourish yourself for the healthiest, happiest life possible—you are a ripe candidate for an attitude adjustment. Some specific techniques for assisting the adjustment process can be found in "Changing Food Attitudes" at the end of this chapter. You will, in effect, be making a shift: food will no longer get star status,

---

3. Many food addicts have found the missing link in their recoveries to be unresolved inner child issues. *Healing the Shame That Binds You* and other works by John Bradshaw can be especially helpful (see Appendix A), along with counseling with sensitive professionals. Certain people have discovered that dealing in therapy with childhood trauma, sometimes trauma buried beneath conscious recall, is necessary before they can maintain consistent abstinence from abusing food. Even more people, however, have found that letting go of food as a drug gives them the clarity and stability they need for the work of deep, inner healing. If you have (or suspect you have) serious, unresolved childhood issues, get the help you need to deal with these as well as your eating problem. Growth in one area can only encourage growth in another.

either as a hero or a villain. It will instead play an important but low-key supporting role.

You are in the ideal place for allowing your attitudes toward food to change because you have been working from the inside out, looking at yourself first, then at your food. Dr. Dean Ornish, author of *Dr. Dean Ornish's Program for Reversing Heart Disease*, uses with his heart patients, many of whom come to him overweight as well, an approach that includes the spiritual disciplines of yoga and meditation, group support, aerobic exercise, and a lowfat, vegetarian diet. He explains the role of inner change in this way:

> It's not enough to simply change behaviors without dealing with deeper issues. Telling someone who's lonely and depressed and isolated that by changing their diet they'll live longer isn't very motivating. Who wants to live longer if they feel bad? So we address the emotional and spiritual dimensions of health and illness, not just the physical. When you feel happier and more peaceful, you tend to choose behaviors which are life-enhancing, rather than self-destructive.[4]

There are many kinds of life-enhancing behaviors. We'll discuss a variety of them in Chapter 9, "The Love-Powered Life." Right now, let's focus on choosing life-enhancing foods. Think about this concept a minute. Life-enhancing food should look good. It should smell good. It should be appealing in its own right. Just because some food is low-calorie or supposedly good for you doesn't necessarily qualify it as life-enhancing. Do you have any childhood memories of having to eat liver or cooked spinach or something else you detested? You may have swallowed it and ingested some useful nutrients in the process, but it's doubtful that you felt your life had been enhanced.

My friend Suzanne is an inspiration when it comes to life-enhancing foods. After she changed her attitudes through spiritual principles, she set about changing her food attitudes most decisively. She cleaned out her kitchen and got rid of everything that didn't add to the health of her body or the beauty of her cupboards. Most of the packaged snack foods went, along with the white sugar and bleached flour. She filled her shelves with tawny grains and colorful beans

---

4. This quote was obtained during a telephone interview with the author (October 1990). Ornish's book is also replete with wisdom, not only for people with heart disease but for the rest of us. See Appendix A.

stored in handsome apothecary jars she'd discovered at a yard sale. Fresh fruit was always ripening on her table or counters, and after she befriended an organic gardener, she learned to grow sprouts, and dry apples, and to notice sunrises, sunsets, and the phases of the moon. She started making juices from concord grapes and from sweet carrots, and creating thick shakes that tasted like rich chocolate malteds[5] but were actually nourishing, satisfying breakfasts. And my friend who had already been beautiful to those who knew her became strikingly so to everyone she met. Her eyes seemed bluer than they'd been before. Her skin seemed translucent. Her body responded to this VIP treatment with glowing health and increased energy.

We influence each other more than we know. This friend and I now have a continent between us, but whenever I'm tempted to throw something together instead of lovingly preparing fresh food, I think of her. Then the need to rush doesn't seem as pressing. I put away the can opener and get out the paring knife.

There is no single, rigid way to eat that is right for everyone. We have different activity levels and different ethnic backgrounds. We live in different climates and in different social environments. Nevertheless, we are physiologically very similar. Based on that similarity, there are guidelines about eating that apply to humans as a species. It makes sense, for instance, to eat primarily the foods that come to us from nature rather than expecting the body to deal with synthetic substances it doesn't understand.

It is known, too, that a diet high in animal fats is the foremost contributor to heart disease, the number one killer in this country. It has also been linked with several kinds of cancer, diabetes, osteoporosis, and many other plagues of civilization, overweight included. People who choose natural foods that are low in fat are healthier, as a rule, than those who eat processed and high-fat foods. Their bodies are leaner, although they eat heartily. In parts of the world where this style of eating is the norm, obesity is virtually unknown. Recovering food addicts who eat in this way do not have to be concerned about their

5. These simple shakes may be made from two ripe bananas (one freshly peeled, one peeled, chopped, and frozen overnight), 3/4 cup of cold water, and 1 teaspoon carob powder (this provides the chocolate taste—get carob powder at a natural food store) and blend. You can find more healthy food preparation ideas in Chapter 8 and Appendix B.

weight, about portion sizes, or cutting back after weekends or holidays.

Combining a spiritual turnaround and this gentle way of eating brings the Love-powered approach full circle. Spirituality is the inner side; gentle, natural, Love-powered food choices the outer. Certainly not everyone who recovers from food addiction by spiritual means chooses the eating style that will be detailed in the following chapters. However, those who do find that it supports and complements their total way of living. It is also amazingly easy. To quote Dr. Ornish:

> On most diets, people count calories and limit portion sizes. They end up feeling hungry so diets don't last and they gain back the weight they lost. Within these guidelines, however, you can eat whenever you're hungry and still lose weight because the food is so low in fat. The result is a sense of abundance rather than deprivation. It's not even a diet, it's a new way of eating.[6]

It may well be that a new way of life deserves—and perhaps demands—a new way of eating. Explore your options. Experiment. Read the books in Appendix A. Use your head. Consult your heart. Talk with your doctor, with your friends, with your God. Your spiritual awakening will provide you with the gift of choice. Unwrap it.

- - - - - - - - - - - - - - - -

◀ THE NOW CHOICE ▶

We can accept the gift of choice only in the present moment. Certainly our lives are enriched by happy memories and fond hopes. We can learn from the past and we must plan for the future, but we're asking for trouble when we try to live in either one. Focusing on the past invites regret and remorse. Denying the present for the future asks for worry and anxiety. Why? Because neither the past nor the future is real. The only reality is this moment. Some people call this "the eternal now."

We are thoroughly in the present when we are engrossed in a proj-

6. Telephone interview with the author, October 1990.

ect and lose track of time. That's when we aren't judging ourselves, when we're not late or early, too young or too old, when we're not concerned about what we've eaten or how much we weigh or anything else. We are in the process of being alive. In even a long life, the hours of being fully, blissfully alive can be few indeed. For many people, most in-the-now time is enjoyed during childhood. Children are grounded in the present to a degree that can be unnerving to adults.

In recovery, we can reclaim a degree of this childlikeness in allowing ourselves to be thoroughly in the present. This concept is particularly important for people who have had problems with food. Food addiction includes a chronic neglect of the present, replacing the attention that today deserves with focusing on last year's thinness or next week's diet. I'm partial to the line in the Lord's Prayer that says, "Give us this day our daily bread." The emphasis is mine because my problem was an unwillingness to gratefully accept my daily bread: I wanted several days' bread with honey and butter and cheese.

Living in the now is one way to come to know through and through that this day's bread—and time and inspiration and whatever else I need—is here for me today. For today, I'm taken care of. So are you.

Growth in recovery is a daily proposition. We can no more live on yesterday's spirituality than on yesterday's oxygen. We claim today's spirituality by making the now choice, by choosing to remember that:

· This is the only moment there is.

· This is the only moment that we have access to our Higher Power.

· This is the only moment we can refrain from eating for a fix and this is the only moment we need to.

◄ CHANGING FOOD ATTITUDES: ►
SOME ACTIONS TO TAKE

1. Allow an inner transformation to take place through bringing your spiritual life to bear on your life as a whole—eating included. Using the Twelve Steps is one proven way to do this.

2. Find at least one person (preferably a group of people) with whom you can talk about your attitudes toward food. Do so

whenever you need to. As soon as you're able, provide the same sort of support for others.

3. Bring your Higher Power into food situations with you. You are not alone when you remember that the God of your understanding is with you all the time. This help is not only available in dramatic situations but at banquets, buffets, and when you're passing a bakery window.

4. Be grateful for your food. Say a prayer of thanks at meals. Remember the contribution of everyone from the earthworms to the farmers, the retailer to the cook (even if that's you).

5. Select and prepare your foods lovingly. Think about what it means to serve food to yourself and others. You are providing physical substance that will become a part of your living body and the bodies of people you care about. You deserve the best and so do they. This is a sacred trust.

6. Choose beautiful food and present it beautifully. Your tongue may prefer fudge to strawberries, but your eyes are partial to strawberries. Indulge them for a change. Experience your meals with all your senses. Eat slowly. Put flowers on the table and play soft music—not just for company, for you.

7. Discover the clean delight of simple food. I remember the first time I had a cup of tea without lemon or cream or sweetener. I was amazed at how delicately flavorful it was, how interesting to taste something I'd drunk many times before without really experiencing it. You can discover something similar with an unbuttered potato, a plain bowl of oatmeal, or air-popped corn. Food certainly doesn't have to be bland or dull, but it is curious that for people who supposedly love food, we don't actually know what most of it tastes like.

8. Learn to feel safe between meals. Sit with the feeling of not being full the way you have learned to sit with other feelings. Don't get spartan about it (that's the dieter's mentality or even the anorexic's) but get to know how it feels to not be digesting food all the time, to know that you can be content without being full.

9. Conversely, experience fullness. It's easy to ignore the body's signals that say "enough." Some people think that the bodies of

chronic overeaters don't even produce these signals anymore, but I believe they're simply ignored. Listen for them. How does it feel to be full? You know, you're okay after a meal and you're okay before one. It's all right to have a full stomach or an empty one. All humans and nonhuman animals at times have one, at times the other. Join the biosphere!

10. *Explore the world around you.* Thinking about eating and thinking about not eating have taken up enough valuable time. It's a wonderland out there! What do you really want to do: take acting lessons, learn to knit, play golf, work for a cause, speak Italian, write short stories? Do it—not after you've had something to eat and not after you lose ten pounds. Do it now.

◄ BEFORE YOU CHOOSE YOUR FOODS ►

Before you choose your foods, make this choice: Choose to love yourself with the food you eat. Many food addicts say, "When I was growing up, food meant love in my house," and use that to rationalize overeating today. There's a hole in the reasoning, though. Maybe love was expressed to you as a child through food, but if you're abusing food now, you're abusing yourself at the same time. There's no love in that.

Decide to love yourself with how you eat just as you're learning to love yourself with how you live. Some of the suggestions coming up will seem familiar. You've heard similar ones before. You may have even tried them. What's different this time, though, is that you are now engaged in a transformative process that is spiritual and thereby total. That transformation will make it possible for you to implement these suggestions, even if you have tried them and failed in the past. In fact, as your inner transformation continues, you'll see that you will be taking many of these measures without giving them any thought. You will read this list and say, "Yes, I'm doing that."

Eat without guilt. *Guilt enjoys its own company. The guiltier you feel, the more you're likely to continue the guilt-producing behavior.*

Eat for your health. *Don't pass this one by because it seems so obvious. How many people do you know who truly choose their foods to bring about high-level health? Precious few. Be one of them.*

Eat slowly. *Even if you only have half an hour for lunch, you don't have to bolt your food. Chew it. Taste it. If your meals are routinely rushed or interrupted (if you work on call, or if you're the parent of small children), make a special point of slowing down for the meals at which you do have that luxury.*

Eat when you're calm and centered. *If you're upset, don't eat, even if it's mealtime. Pray. Take a walk or a bath. Phone someone. Sane eating and inner turmoil are rarely found at the same table.*

Eat the way that's best for you, regardless of others' opinions. *The majority of people are far superior to the food they eat. Every human being is a divine creation entitled to the very best, yet most people in our culture eat quantities of fast, fragmented, and foodless food. When you stop joining them in this, they're liable to rib you about being a health nut or being on some foolish diet. You need to remember that you're neither and continue to do what's right for you.*

Eat food prepared with love, care, and attention. *When you are the chef, prepare your foods in this way. When you eat out, choose places where you are most likely to get food that had love, care, and attention given it. This doesn't have to mean always going to expensive restaurants. Those places that prepare their foods fresh, that are privately owned and have the owners on the premises, those that specialize in natural foods, and many ethnic restaurants (particularly family businesses) are as concerned with these intangibles as with the special of the day.*

Allow your tastes and preferences to change for the better. *When you are committed to treating yourself well with the food you eat, you are willing to make some changes, to try some new things. You probably won't like all of them and you don't need to, but you can allow your tastes and preferences to change, to appreciate new textures, subtle flavors, lighter versions of dishes that couldn't offer you the love you deserve.*

Let your food choices express who you are. *You are a beautiful, healthy, compassionate, intelligent human being. You can select foods that are beautiful to look at, smell, and taste; that contribute to the health of your body; that express compassion to others; and that are the result of intelligent discernment.*

These suggestions can more easily become a part of your thinking and thereby a part of your life if you turn them into affirmations.

1. *I eat in love, not in guilt.*

2. *I eat for high-level health.*

3. *I eat slowly. There is plenty of time.*

4. *I eat only when I am calm and centered (or) I give myself the gift of becoming centered before every meal.*

5. *I eat the way that is best for me, regardless of anyone else's opinion.*

6. *I eat only food prepared with love, care, and attention (or, when you're cooking) I prepare this food with love, care, and attention.*

7. *I allow my tastes and preferences to change for the better.*

8. *I let my food choices express who I am (or) I make food choices that express beauty, healthfulness, intelligence, and compassion.*

-❈❈-

SIX

The

Love-Powered

Diet

I feel like an anchorperson on one of the morning news shows in saying, "If you've just joined us . . ." but I know the urge to skip the pre-
liminaries and go straight to the diet. If you're starting here instead of
at the beginning, welcome. You're soon to discover a lifesaving and
life-affirming way of eating that will do your body good while it sends
feelings of deprivation packing. Diet cannot, however, cure a food addict any more than drugs can cure a drug addict. It will take more than
an eating plan to heal the emotional wounds you may have tried to
salve with food. It is critical that you learn to live in conscious contact

with the Love that is able to give you the emotional strength no diet can provide. The first five chapters of this book discuss Love and how to reshape yourself from the inside out.

Nevertheless, if you prefer to start reading here, by all means do. The power of Love is expressed in a practical manner through the way of eating introduced in this chapter, and when that power touches you anywhere, it touches you everywhere. You can begin here, looking at loving food choices, and then you will want to go back and learn about the entire spiritual process. In this case, wanting to have it all isn't greed; it's good sense.

Now, what on earth could Love (which you may call God, Goddess, Higher Power, Nature, Spirit, or something else) have to do with what you eat? Chances are it hasn't had much to do with it, and that put you in the pickle that led you to this book. Surely no loving God and no loving part of yourself wants you tormented by food cravings, subjected to depressing and even dangerous diets, or risking your life with morbid obesity or a binge/purge merry-go-round that ceases to be merry long before the ride is over. It also stands to reason that a loving God or your most loving self would be interested in your overall welfare and the welfare of all people, all forms of life, and of an earth so nurturing to us that many call her mother.

Because Love encompasses everything, nothing is unimportant, including tonight's dinner menu. Think about it for a minute: if you were pure Love, the loving Parent of all life, how would you want people to eat? I wish I could hear your answer. Perhaps you would want people to nourish themselves in a way that:

· Is generous, delicious, and aesthetically pleasing
· Promotes high-level health as well as normal weight
· Is economical and provides plenty for everybody
· Respects all life
· Is environmentally sustainable

We have just described the Love-powered diet.

Truly diet can be a four-letter word and sentences like, "I'm a fat slob and ought to go on a diet" or "I was bad and blew my diet," are no less than obscene. I'm using the word quite differently here. The Love-powered diet applies to a natural, gentle style of eating that uses the D-word in its general and nonthreatening sense, as when you say, "I make sure my children get a balanced diet." What people eat is their *diet*. Depriving oneself in order to lose weight is *dieting*.

There is no dieting here and no menus, no amounts, and no absolutes. Why should I tell you what to eat on some hypothetical Days one through seven as if you had only a week to live? You have a *life* to live, and it isn't hypothetical. Besides, in real life every day is Day one. At this point in your progress along the continuum of inner to outer well-being, you're ready for recommendations, not regimentation. You don't need rules to resist but tools to get new concepts off the drawing board and into practice.

To that end, we'll explore in detail the dietary part of the Love-powered life. We'll first discuss what there is to eat (a lot) and some caveats that, when respected, will help you attain and maintain the slim, healthy body you want. Then we'll look at the Love-powered diet in relation to those five points that you and I decided comprise a loving way of eating.

The Love-powered diet celebrates the abundance of nature. Its basic food groups are:

- Fruits—preferably fresh, also frozen unsweetened
- Vegetables—raw in salads and as crudités, also steamed, sautéed, baked (potatoes fit here, too)
- Whole grains—breads, pastas, and cereal grains like rice and oats
- Legumes—dried beans, peas, lentils, and soy foods such as tofu and tempeh[1]

There is also an auxiliary category of "rich relatives." These foods are higher in oil content or in natural sugars than the basic foods are. They are used in smaller quantities as condiments or garnishes and also to supplement the diet of people who need extra calories to maintain their weight. Rich relatives include: nuts and seeds (preferably raw and unsalted), olives, avocado, and extra-virgin olive oil;[2] and

---

1. Soy products are higher in fat content than other basic Love-powered foods. People who require or prefer a very, very lowfat way of eating can treat them as rich relatives.
2. All vegetable oils are equally concentrated and should be used sparingly when necessary and eliminated when possible.

dried fruits, fruit juices, all-fruit jam, and sweeteners such as honey, sorghum, and pure maple syrup.

All this translates into meals such as fruit plates, fruit smoothies (luscious blender shakes), crisp salads, vegetable stir-fries, casseroles and chowders, hearty whole wheat bread and yummy quick loaves like cornbread and banana bread, an assortment of rice and noodle dishes, Boston baked beans, and satisfying soups such as lentil and split pea. The world of ethnic cooking comes alive for Love-powered chefs, too. You can experiment with dishes from

The Middle East
pita bread sandwiches with hummus (chickpea spread) or baba ganoush (eggplant dip), tabouli (cracked wheat salad), rice pilafs

Italy
spaghetti, fettucine, linguini, even lasagna and pizza made without meats and cheeses that are high in fat

India
a variety of vegetable curries with tantalizing complementary chutneys, dal (spicy sauces made from lentils or split peas), pungent rice dishes

Mexico
chili sans carne, avocado tostadas, bean burritos, taco salad

France
crepes, delicately seasoned Parisian vegetables, and quiche (yes, you can make quiche without eggs, cheese, or cream—and without all their fat and cholesterol)[3]

Even traditional American fare like burgers can be prepared using lowfat, vegetarian recipes. You can create wonderful substitutes for familiar foods so you won't think about what you're no longer eating. Chapter 8 has details on food selection and preparation, and dining out. You'll see that a Love-powered diet is infinitely flexible. You can customize it to fit the way *you* live.

If you don't quite believe that, it's probably because of a single word

---

3. A quiche recipe is included in Appendix B, "Cookbooks and Selected Recipes."

in the preceding paragraph: vegetarian. It is true that the Love-powered diet, when followed completely, is vegetarian. In fact, because it includes no foods of animal origin, it is a total vegetarian or vegan (VEEgun) plan. Stay with me on this, and let me reassure you that eating primarily from the plant kingdom—most of the time or even all of the time—will not change your politics, your religion, or any other part of yourself that the label "vegetarian" doesn't seem to fit. You never need to use the word if you're not comfortable with it, and because the Love-powered diet doesn't require *absolute* adherence, you can make progress without becoming strictly vegetarian. In his book *The McDougall Plan*, John McDougall, M.D., suggests a low-fat vegan diet, but he allows healthy people the option of including some other things on occasion as "feast foods." This might work for you, too. And after reading the list of famous vegetarians of the past and present at the end of this chapter, you'll see that if you do decide to go all the way with this, you'll be in good company.

You've probably already deduced that the Love-powered diet doesn't just bypass animal foods, it leaves out most of the highly refined, overprocessed, phony foods we're fond of calling junk. The majority of items found in convenience stores and gas stations, much of what's in an ordinary bakery, and probably everything at the movie theater except lightly salted popcorn is junk food. The supermarket has its share of nutritionally vacant items, and some of them can even creep into a health food store. Reading labels is a good practice, but the best food is usually fresh food—no package, no label.

For the Love-powered diet to give you all it can, you'll want to avoid any food that isn't good enough for you—just the way your mother told you not to date Sammy Smith for that very reason. If it's high in sugar (when sugar is near the top of an ingredients list, that's high), high in salt (enough to make you thirsty), or very fatty (if it's fried, "melts in your mouth," or leaves a shine on a napkin)—well, meet Sammy Smith.

❧ A TASTE FOR QUALITY ❧

Everyone knows that junk food is a nutritional disaster, packs in the calories, and causes a yen for more of the same. In addition, it simply isn't becoming to someone who's out to love himself or herself more.

You can go to an elegant restaurant and consume a thousand calories in a special dinner with a special person, and leave there feeling super about the world and everything that's in it—yourself included. Or you could go to some fast food place, gobble up a thousand calories in 4.2 minutes and feel fat and guilty as you toss the wrappers. Cultivate your taste for quality and select the best food you can afford.

Go for quality drinks, too, since many are questionable. Alcohol, with its empty calories and mood-altering potential, should be saved for moderate consumption on special occasions, if you choose to drink at all. A typical soft drink contains some nine teaspoons of sugar in a twelve-ounce can, and all artificial sweeteners are still controversial.[4]

The caffeine in cola, as well as in coffee and tea, can also be a problem. Caffeine is a drug, a stimulant. The easiest way to modify a caffeine induced "buzz" is to eat, and many people do this unconsciously. Caffeine can also suppress the appetite temporarily, but it comes back like gangbusters. Dieters usually drink lots of coffee, tea, and cola, and dieters usually relapse. It's possible that there is a caffeine connection. According to Agatha Thrash, M.D., "Any drug that will stimulate the nerves will stimulate the appetite in susceptible people. This includes coffee, tea, colas, and chocolate. These beverages stimulate cravings."[5]

If you consume beverages that contain caffeine, pay attention to the ways they affect your attitude, and your appetite. You may decide to discontinue or moderate your use and try herbal teas, sparkling mineral water, and natural spritzers (mineral water and fruit juice) instead. The drink that helped get a diet cola hankering the size of Texas off my back is licorice tea. Hot or iced, this herbal is naturally sweet but calorically negligible.

With animal products, junk foods and iffy drinks out of your diet, you will also have inadvertently eliminated all or most of your per-

4. Regarding aspartame (NutraSweet): "There is no convincing evidence that this chemical helps control weight, and it is implicated in convulsions and other nervous system problems . . . children and pregnant women are strongly advised to avoid it, and that is good advice for everyone else as well." Neal Bernard, M.D., *The Power of Your Plate*, p. 80. See Appendix A.
5. Agatha Thrash, M.D., *Nutrition for Vegetarians* (Seale, AL: New Lifestyle Books, 1982), p. 122.

sonal binge foods. You may, however, have others and it's important that you come to terms with them. Not everyone who wants to lose a few pounds has binge foods, but if you've ever been on an eating binge—that's a drunk that you chew—you're probably intimately acquainted with them. I've heard them described as "better than sex" and "one bite is too many and a thousand aren't enough." These are the foods that encourage appetite instead of extinguishing it. You really *can't* eat just one. If you have some today, you'll need more tomorrow. In other words, binge foods are addictive.

The usual recipe for a binge food is fat plus sugar or fat plus salt. Common culprits, then, are what you'd expect: ice cream, chips, chocolate, pastries, cheese. But even something as subtle as combining nuts and raisins for trail mix can turn two otherwise innocuous foods into the makings of some overeater's lost weekend. Besides, binge foods are intensely personal. For a given individual, something about the taste or texture of almost any food, or past associations with it, can make it far more than just something to eat. You may have trouble with a broad general category—sugar, meat, flour, anything at your mom's house—or specific items: granola, yogurt, dates, peanut butter, white bread.

If you can be really honest with yourself, you'll probably realize that you already know your own red-light foods. You may not want to claim them, but you may as well; they've already claimed you. If you're unsure about a specific suspect, try to eat a little and save the rest for a week from Thursday. If you can't do it, or if you think incessantly about *it* in the cupboard or fridge, you've got yourself a binge food.

The point in identifying these is to protect you from infiltrators out to sabotage your victory. If you had an enemy who was set on harming you, you would do everything in your power to protect yourself. You would notify the police and obtain a restraining order to keep him or her away from your house! Understand that any food you haven't been able to eat reasonably since you cut teeth is as threatening to you as that enemy. The safest path to tread with a binge food is the one that leads away from it. In other words, don't eat it—not because I said so, but because you would rather not socialize with a dietary hit man.

The prospect of living without some food you've depended on can seem unbearable, but you can do it. The secret is to think in terms of *today* instead of eternity. There is disagreement among eating disorder experts and recovering overeaters (who are also experts in my opinion) on whether or not these dynamite foods can ever be defused. That is to say, can the allure of carrot cake come down to that of carrot sticks? I've found that I'm able to eat anything that I choose to eat *today providing it is appropriate*. This means that I'll have cake at a birthday party, but I don't keep cakes around to call to me the way the sirens sang to those ancient Greek sailors.

With what the Twelve Step Programs call HOW—honesty, open-mindedness, and willingness—you'll find your own way with binge foods. They are potentially loaded weapons, but as you live by Love-powered principles, they'll lose much of their attraction. One of these days, you'll find yourself looking at a onetime temptation as if it were an old flame and thinking, "What did I ever see in that one?"

Snacking—snacking with wild abandon at least—can meet a similar fate. With the Love-powered diet, you can elect to snack on something that will support your health and your progress, or you may decide not to snack. Every so often, some study reports that eating small, frequent meals (snacking or "grazing") is superior to having three regular meals. This works for certain people and there are, in fact, medical conditions which require it. For most of us, though, the sanest approach is also the simplest: three reasonable meals a day, eaten on a fairly predictable schedule.

In the earliest stages of your lifestyle change, you may need *large* meals to bridge the gap between binge-eating and moderation. That's fine. Begin wherever you can. With a basic commitment to three meals, you'll find that, in starting to eat only three times, you have to *stop* only three times. For anyone with a food or weight problem, stopping was always the hard part. Moreover, society is set up for three meals a day. You go on vacation and stay at a bed and breakfast. Your work day is punctuated with a lunch hour. You're invited out for dinner.

As you embark on your adventure with the Love-powered diet, you'll be enjoying bountiful meals and may well find that three of these a day with nothing but living in between are fully adequate. On the other hand, this is a lowfat food plan which includes lots of water-rich fruits and vegetables that are efficiently processed by your digestive apparatus. They don't stay with you like heavy, fatty foods that must be laboriously digested. Therefore, you may well want something to eat at morning break time, mid-afternoon, or before bed. *The best snack is a piece of fruit.* This is the original, portable fast food. The natural sugars in fruit will pick up your energy, and it's as close to fat-free as you're going to get.

Have fruit between meals if you want it. Raw vegetables make good snacks, too, although they can seem too much like diet food for some. In any event, you never have to be hungry. You may at times *choose* to feel hungry; and that's all right, too. Oh, I know that no book like this is supposed to suggest that you'll ever feel any less satiated than a just-nursed infant, but that isn't realistic. Mom doesn't pack us lunches anymore, and there will be times that we'd like to eat and will need to wait. Saying no sometimes is as much a part of the privilege of adulthood as saying yes.

This is where flexibility comes in, flexibility of your food plan and of your thinking. When you or I are in "fit spiritual condition,"[6] we can make rational decisions, even when those decisions are about food. Let's say you have to dash to the airport without having supper, and the kiosk near your flight gate only has candy bars and salted peanuts. You have a choice. You can buy a candy bar or some peanuts, or you can choose to feel a little hungry and wait until food you'd prefer is available. What would you do? If it were me, I'd go without for the time being if something were to be served on the plane. If, however, I had to wait until I got to Cleveland for my next meal, I would get a bag of peanuts. Even though I don't usually eat salted nuts and generally stick with fruit between meals, this would be a perfectly legitimate action in a less than perfect situation.

There may be some fabled Diet Land where airport newsstands sell celery, and where you can have half a banana today and the other half won't turn brown while you save it for day after tomorrow. I just don't live in a place like that, and I don't think you do either. Around here, it makes more sense to have a whole banana

6. *Alcoholics Anonymous*, p. 85.

and maybe even some peanuts every once in a while. You can do that with Love-powered eating because it's designed to work in the real world, the same world that actively benefits when you choose Love-powered foods. This brings us back to those five points that we came up with at the beginning of this chapter. Let's take a closer look at each one now.

A Love-powered diet is generous, delicious, and aesthetically pleasing. A downside of dieting is lack of food. You're told to compensate by using a smaller plate. Now you can use a standard plate and a *big* salad bowl. If a substantial salad with light, nonoily dressing is the center of your meal, ordinary salad bowls are a joke. Uncooked vegetables as well as fruits are both low in fat and high in water; therefore they are lower in calories. The filling starches from which you'll make most of your entrées—rice, pasta, beans, potatoes (yes, plural!)—are lowfat foods as well, so they're lower in calories than traditional main dishes. In addition, there is some evidence suggesting that calories from fat are actually more fattening than the same number of calories from carbohydrates. Even the leaner animal foods are generally fattier than grains, vegetables, and most beans.[7]

I'm not suggesting that because most Love-powered foods won't put you at odds with the bathroom scale you should overeat. I am saying, however, that the concept of a moderate portion has to be redefined when you adopt a lowfat diet. If you're having salad, steamed asparagus, and corn on the cob for dinner, don't have one ear of corn—have three or four, and a roll besides. And those boxes of rice pilaf don't serve six anymore. They served six with roast beef. As a main course, they'll serve two.

Not only are Love-powered portions generous, the variety of foods from which you'll choose is enormous. When people find out that you're doing this, they'll say, "But what do you eat?" Take it from me: they wouldn't stand still long enough to hear all the marvelous foods on nature's table. The lists in Chapter 8 are just a beginning. When you're eating natural foods and concentrating on those from the plant kingdom, you'll become far more aware of seasonal fruits and vegeta-

---

7. For a more detailed discussion on fats, see Chapter 7.

bles. You will discover regional delights as you travel that are lost to people on the burger-and-fries circuit. There are hundreds of different varieties of vegetables and fruits, dozens of kinds of grains and legumes, and plenty of interesting specialty and convenience foods made from them. From this abundance, you can select what you like. You don't have to eat any specific food—not grapefruit, not spinach, not soybeans. *You* build your eating plan around foods you already like, and with a little daring you can discover both delicious new foods and tasty new ways to fix old favorites.

Either way, what you'll offer yourself and others to eat will *look* beautiful. A supermarket checker once bagged my week's provisions and said, "I've had this job fifteen years and I've never seen such pretty groceries!" That's because fruits and vegetables really are edible works of art, and whether in a shopping cart or on a serving tray, they are very appealing to people. Natural, vegetarian foods entice the eye, and have wonderful fragrances and distinctive flavors. They tantalize several senses, and meals based on them invite appreciation and the slower pace that's essential in retraining eating habits. It's also pleasant to be in the company of these foods. If you were going to meet a friend in the city, wouldn't you rather rendezvous at a fruit stand than at a butcher's shop or fish market? And if you went back to your place for the kind of simple but elegant dinner you will soon be adept at preparing, cleanup would be a breeze. Greasy pots do not exist when you eat a Love-powered diet, and that counts as aesthetically pleasing, too.

A Love-powered diet promotes high-level health as well as normal weight. "I have lived quite long enough and am trying to die," wrote vegetarian George Bernard Shaw at eighty-four, "but I simply cannot do it. A single beefsteak would finish me, but I cannot bring myself to swallow it. I am oppressed with a dread of living forever. That is the only disadvantage of vegetarianism." There isn't any diet, of course, that can substitute for genes programmed for longevity, but a poor diet can keep you from reaching your potential for both quality and length of life."

Chapter 7 is devoted to nutrition and to the many health benefits of lowfat, minimally processed foods from the vegetable kingdom. For now, let me shower you with statistics reported by John Robbins in his book *Diet for a New America* and taken here from the EarthSave booklet *Realities for the 90's.*[8]

The average American man has a 50% chance of dying from heart attack; the average total vegetarian man reduces that risk to 4%.

No country in the world with a high intake of meat has a low incidence of colon cancer.

Women who eat eggs 3 or more days a week compared to less than once a week have a 3 times greater risk of developing fatal ovarian cancer.

Men who consume meats, dairy products, and eggs daily as compared to sparingly run a 3.6 times greater risk of developing fatal prostate cancer.

The average measurable bone loss of female meat eaters at age 65 is 35%; in vegetarian women it is 18%.

According to one study published in the *New England Journal of Medicine*, the chlorinated hydrocarbon pesticide contamination of the average American mother's breast milk is greater than 30 times higher than that of vegetarian nursing mothers'.

A variety of factors may account for the apparent superiority of a vegetarian or near-vegetarian diet. In replacing animal foods with unrefined grains, fruits, vegetables, and legumes, a dietary program results that is:

· Cholesterol-free (the cholesterol in our diet comes *only* from foods of animal origin)
· Low in fats, especially saturated fats
· High in natural carbohydrates
· Rich in fiber
· Abundant in vitamins A and C which some research indicates may protect against certain cancers, as well as other possible anticarcinogens such as indoles in cruciferous (cabbage family) vegetables and protease inhibitors in legumes

8. *Realities for the 90's* is a compilation of facts from *Diet for a New America* by John Robbins. It is available from EarthSave, 706 Frederick Street, Santa Cruz, CA 95062-2205. These statistics come from pp. 4, 5, and 7 of the *Realities for the 90's* booklet.

- Adequate but not excessive in protein (too much protein has been linked with osteoporosis, kidney stones, and deterioration of kidney function)
- Markedly lower in pesticide residues, particularly the chlorinated hydrocarbons like dieldrin and DDT which accumulate in the body fat of animals and humans
- Bulky and satisfying to assuage hunger without excess calories

It is, therefore, widely accepted in the medical literature[9] that vegans, people who eat only plant foods and no meat, fish, eggs, or dairy products, weigh less than omnivores by eight to twenty pounds, depending on the study. The omnivores average seventeen to twenty-two pounds over ideal.[10] **The serendipitous thing about vegans and weight is that their slimness is not something they work at. It happens naturally—without hunger, suffering, or willpower.** That's precisely how it will happen for you provided you practice the spiritual principles that will keep you from needing to eat for a fix, and build your diet from the four Love-powered food groups.

The Love-powered diet is economical and provides plenty for everybody. You can afford a Love-powered diet, even if you're a full-time student, a retired person on a fixed income, or a food stamp recipient. The staples for this eating style are among the most inexpensive foods in the marketplace: rice, beans, whole wheat flour and bread, potatoes, carrots, greens and other seasonal vegetables, apples, oranges, bananas and other fruits selected when they're most abundant and least costly. You'll be saving cash by skipping the high-ticket items like meat and cheese, as well as the junk foods which are only bargains until you consider the physiological price you pay for them.

You certainly can spend money on rare, tropical fruits, exotic vegetables (I'm astounded by how many vegetables come in purple), health food store convenience items, and gourmet specialties. You don't need these, though, to design Love-powered menus that are nutritious and conducive to bringing your best body into being.

9. *American Journal of Clinical Nutrition* 23:249, 1970; *American Journal of Clinical Nutrition* 6:523, 1958; *New England Journal of Medicine* 292:1148, 1975.
10. *Journal Nutrition*, Vol. 10, No. 6, 1963, reported by Nathaniel Altman in *Eating for Life*, p. 150 (New York: Vegetus Books, 1986).

Not only is this way of eating wallet-friendly, it can, in an indirect way at least, help make more food available for more people, notably for the 20,000,000 who, according to the Institute for Food and Development Policy and Oxfam America, die each year as a result of malnutrition. The connection is that raising animals for food uses vast amounts of land and other resources for a meager return in protein and calories. Frances Moore Lappé's landmark book *Diet for a Small Planet*, originally published in 1971, was the first popular work to point this out. The modern habit of feeding grains and soybeans to cattle and other animals destined for slaughter makes the raising of animals for food particularly inefficient. Lappé called these animals "protein factories in reverse" and described how it takes sixteen pounds of grain and soy to produce one pound of feedlot beef, six pounds to produce one pound of pork, and three pounds to produce one pound of chicken or eggs. "To give you some basis for comparison," she wrote, "sixteen pounds of grain has twenty-one times more calories and eight times more protein—but only three times more fat—than a pound of hamburger."[11]

If our meat consumption were reduced by even ten percent, enough land, water, and energy would be freed to raise food for 60,000,000 people; and on a Love-powered diet, fifteen people could be fed from the land needed to feed just one person on typical American fare.[12]

It is simplistic to assume that, given the economic and political realities of the present day, world hunger will be eradicated simply through a dietary change on the part of people in the wealthier nations. Nevertheless, it is not logistically possible to feed the world on the sort of diet we were brought up to believe is normal and necessary, a diet that relies heavily on meat and other animal foods.

If only as a way to stand in solidarity with those who do not have enough, we can decide in our food choices to "live simply that others may simply live." And this can be done without in any way confining ourselves to austerity rations. Simplicity and asceticism are about as

11. Frances Moore Lappé, *Diet for a Small Planet* (quote, p. 69, conversion ratios from Fig. 1, p. 70, "A Protein Factory in Reverse," statistics from USDA, Economic Research Service, Beltsville, MD). This comes from the 10th Anniversary Edition of *Diet for a Small Planet* (New York: Ballantine Books, 1982).
12. From EarthSave booklet *Realities for the 90's*, p. 2.

closely related as cabbages and cocker spaniels. Simple foods, those that the earth provides generously for all, can be the makings of elegant repasts, celebrations of life and health in good taste and good conscience.

A Love-powered diet respects all life. In summer and fall, the classifieds are filled with ads for "Pik-Ur-Own" places, inviting city folks on a country outing that will bring in a miniature harvest of apples or berries. That's the same time of year that the gardeners are out in force, turning suburban yards into small truck farms or greening midtown balconies with lettuce and radish and tomato plants. People delight in these pursuits, even before the fruits of their labors reach the dining table.

Throughout the year, however, something else is going on. Animals are being slaughtered for meat, not a few but nearly *six billion* a year in the United States alone. (If a billion is a difficult figure to comprehend, consider that a million seconds pass in eleven and one-half days; for a billion seconds to pass takes nearly thirty-two years![13]) We usually don't stop to think that a Kansas City steak was recently a Kansas cow, but as philosopher Peter Singer wrote in his book *Animal Liberation*, "For most humans, especially those in modern urban and suburban communities, the most direct form of contact with nonhuman animals is at meal time: we eat them."[14]

Many people believe that this is just as it should be and it certainly isn't my place to meddle in your personal ethics. You need not be a vegetarian to develop the spiritual connection that will free you from the need to abuse food. Maintaining that connection does, however, ask that we take responsibility for our actions. Would you, in an ordinary, nonemergency situation, kill an animal and eat it? Most people find the prospect repulsive—quite unlike picking apples or growing tomato plants.

In fact, most people I know who support with their food choices the killing of animals for meat refuse to tour a slaughterhouse. I asked fifteen of them, and none would go. I went by myself. There was a

13. I did not figure this out on my abacus. It's from a book, *Innumeracy: Mathematical Illiteracy and Its Consequences*, by John Allen Paulos (NY: Hill and Wang, 1988).
14. Peter Singer, *Animal Liberation, a New Ethics for Our Treatment of Animals* (New York: Avon Books, 1990), p. 92.

particular cow I will always remember. She was old, a reject from a dairy herd; "used up," the man said. She seemed used to people, and trusting, so she didn't require the cattle prod—an instrument that is capable of producing first-degree burns—to walk the ramp to the metal enclosure where she would be stunned with the captive bolt pistol. When the worker came at her with the stunner, she crouched to avoid it. He *whistled* at her, the way I imagined he might whistle at his dog when he got home that evening. She raised her head in response, was shot with the captive bolt, dropped to the kill floor, and within minutes was unceremoniously transformed from being to beef. "You have just dined," wrote Emerson, "and however scrupulously the slaughterhouse is concealed in the distance of miles, there is complicity."

Unlike in Emerson's day, though, there is a problem in the barnyard as well as at the abattoir. Most of the animals raised for food today come from factory farms where they may be confined to small cages or stalls, and are dehorned, detailed, debeaked, and mutilated in other ways. Many are denied exercise, companionship, natural diets, and other basic needs, and there are no federal laws protecting them.

Calves raised for milk-fed veal are separated from their mothers soon after birth and sent to live their sixteen-week lives chained by the neck in crates too small for them to turn around in. They are given no bedding—they might eat it and obtain iron that would adulterate their white flesh—and they are fed an antibiotic-laced liquid diet, designed to cause anemia and guarantee white meat. It's common to keep the calves in total darkness, and many are blind when they reach the slaughterhouse. Lots of people who are aware of this system boycott milk-fed veal and restaurants that serve it, but not all these people realize that the *raison d'être* of the veal industry is the dairy industry. Veal calves are the superfluous males from dairy herds. Some people do not use dairy products for this reason.

Hens involved in egg production have an unsavory life as well. Male chicks are culled at birth and killed. This spares them the fate of their sisters who will mature into laying hens and spend all their productive lives crammed in tiny, stacked cages with so many birds that none can walk or spread even one wing. The elaborate social system (pecking order) of the chickens is thwarted and they resort to so-called vices such as cannibalism. To minimize this, they are debeaked—a painful process involving cutting sensitive tissue with a hot knife. Instincts like scratching the earth, dustbathing, nest-building, mating, being part of a flock, and experiencing the outdoors are denied. After nine months or so, the hens are slaughtered for soup or potpies. It is possible to obtain free-range eggs from a farmer you know or, at a premium price, from some health food stores or the occasional supermarket. Another option is to refrain from eating eggs.[15]

Consideration for the animals involved may never be your motivation for a diet that excludes animal foods. Still, expect that as you adopt some of the principles found here your overall reverence for life will expand. You may not interpret or express that reverence in the way that someone else might, but expect to see it in your life because it will be there. As psychologist Virginia Satir wrote, "Spiritual power can be seen in a person's reverence for life—hers and all others, including animals and nature, with a recognition of a universal life force referred to by many as God."

A Love-powered diet is environmentally sustainable. It is as gentle to the earth as it is to animals and arteries. For this reason, the bestselling *50 Simple Things You Can Do to Save the Earth*, which ushered in the environmental decade of the 1990s, includes as one of its suggestions, "Eat Low on the Food Chain."[16] Curiously, it's included in the book's final section labeled "For the Committed." In practice, eating low on the food chain (following the Love-powered diet or one similar to it) can be just as easy to incorporate into an ecologically aware lifestyle as other responsible practices like recycling cans and recharging batteries.

Why a diet that does not depend on animal foods is vital in restoring health to an ailing planet is explained in the following facts and figures from John Robbins:

> 75% of U.S. topsoil has been lost to date, and 85% of U.S. topsoil loss is directly associated with livestock raising.

15. To read more about the condition of animals in modern intensive agriculture, see *Animal Factories: An Inside Look at Manufacturing Food for Profit*, by Jim Mason and Peter Singer (NY: Crown Publishers, 1990).
16. The EarthWorks Group, *50 Simple Things You Can Do to Save the Earth*, p. 46 (listed in Appendix A).

260,000,000 acres of U.S. forests have been cleared for cropland to produce a meat-centered diet.

Every individual who switches to a complete vegetarian diet saves an acre of trees each year.

33% of all raw materials (base products of farming, forestry, and mining, including fossil fuels) consumed by the U.S. are devoted to the production of livestock.

More than half the water used for *all purposes* in the United States goes for livestock production.

Livestock in this country produce 230,000 pounds of excrement *every second*. Feedlots do not have sewage systems, so with every rainstorm a part of the 1 billion tons of waste generated annually in confinement operations goes into streams, rivers, and groundwater.

A driving force behind the destruction of tropical rain forests is the American meat habit.

To get a single calorie of protein from beef requires seventy-eight calories of fossil fuel; a calorie of protein from soybeans requires just two calories of fossil fuel.[17]

Statistics can be numbing and the whole notion of an environmental crisis can seem so overwhelming that the very thought of it can push a shut-off valve in our psyches to divert our thinking elsewhere. True, the earth's ills are enormous and it will take action on myriad fronts to heal them. Contributing to the well-being of the planet with earth-loving food choices is one such action, one which takes no time and no extraordinary effort. You're probably busy with all sorts of things, but you will stop for lunch, and making it a Love-powered meal can be an effortless donation to a most deserving planet.[18]

In addition to the environmental benefits brought about by eating

17. These figures come from *Realities for the 90's* and from a lecture given by Robbins at the North American Vegetarian Society "Summerfest," Allentown, Pennsylvania, 1988.
18. Books which go into detail about the environmental effects of our food choices include *Diet for a New America* by John Robbins (see Appendix A), and *A Vegetarian Sourcebook* by Keith Akers (P.O. Box 61273, Denver, CO 80206: Vegetarian Press, 1989).

low on the food chain, there are subtler ways in which a Love-powered diet supports an eco-ethic. Since you'll be selecting natural foods, many of which can be purchased in bulk and put in reusable containers, you'll be using fewer packaging materials. You'll be less likely to frequent fast food places with their plethora of disposables, and since you will not have meat scraps, all your garbage can be composted if you're so inclined. With some of the money you save, you can buy some food organically grown, and with more fresh fruits and salads in your diet, you may use your stove less often and save energy. Also, this is clean eating. With it, you will have fewer dishes to wash so you won't need as much detergent or hot water.

Trying a Love-powered diet may cause the environmentalist within you to emerge since you will be inviting nature right into your kitchen. Don't be surprised if you find yourself growing parsley and chives in clay pots on your window sills, or raising a continuous crop of alfalfa sprouts on the counter by the sink. You might even find yourself planting a tree that, in a few years or several, will bear fruit or nuts. When this was first suggested to me, I argued. "Why should I plant a fruit tree? I won't even be living in this house when it gets its first peach." "Someone will be living there," I was reminded. A tree, then, can be a contribution to strangers and the earth.

And eating from trees and gardens and fields can be a gift to yourself, one of all sorts of ways you'll discover to make the love in your life practical and viable. "Love is a force," wrote Anne Morrow Lindbergh. "It is not a result; it is a cause. It is not a product; it produces. It is a power, like money, or steam or electricity. It is valueless unless you can give something else by means of it."[19] With a Love-powered diet, you give a great deal, and you get even more in return.

19. Anne Morrow Lindbergh, quoted in Anonymous, *Each Day a New Beginning, Daily Meditations for Women* (Center City, MN: Hazelden, 1982), August 16.

SOME FAMOUS VEGETARIANS OF THE PAST AND PRESENT

Philosophy and Religion

Buddha	*Porphyry*
Clement of Alexandria	*Pythagoras*
Ralph Waldo Emerson	*Peter Singer*
Stephen Gaskin	*Henry David Thoreau*
J. Krishnamurti	*John Wesley*
Plato	*Ellen G. White*

Literature & Journalism

Louisa May Alcott	*George Bernard Shaw*
Laura Huxley	*Percy Bysshe Shelley*
Colman McCarthy	*Isaac Bashevis Singer*
John Milton	*Rabindranath Tagore*
Malcolm Muggeridge	*Leo Tolstoy*

Science & Medicine

Max Bircher-Benner	*John Harvey Kellogg*
Charles Darwin	*Isaac Newton*
Albert Einstein	*Albert Schweitzer*
Sylvester Graham	*Leonardo da Vinci*

Politics & Social Reform

Susan B. Anthony	*Cesar Chavez*
Clara Barton	*Mahatma Gandhi*
Annie Besant	*Horace Greeley*
General William Booth	*Helen and Scott Nearing*

Sports

Ridgely Abele (World Championship, Karate)

Peter Burwash (Canadian champion & Davis Cup star, tennis)

Andreas Cahling (Mr. International, bodybuilding)

James & Jonathan deDonato
(world records, distance butterfly stroke, swimming)

Ruth Heidrich (Ironman triathlete)

Kathy Johnson (Olympic gymnast)

Tony LaRussa (manager, Oakland Athletics baseball team)

Sixto Linares (world record holder, 24-hour triathalon—4.8 miles
swimming, 185 miles cycling, 52.5 miles running)

Edwin Moses (undefeated 8 years in 400-meter hurdles)

Bess Motta ("20 Minute Workout," aerobics)

Gayle Olinekova (marathoner)

Bill Pearl (4-time Mr. Universe, bodybuilding)

Bill Pickering (world record, swimming English Channel)

Stan Price (world record, bench press, weight lifting)

Murray Rose
(world records, 400- & 1500-meter freestyle, swimming)

Susan Smith-Jones, Ph.D. (professor, physical education)

Entertainment

Meredith Baxter-Birney	River Phoenix
Jeff Beck	Phylicia Rashad
Ellen Burstyn	Fred "Mister" Rogers
Julie Christie	Ravi Shankar
Dick Gregory	Sting
Michael Jackson	Cicily Tyson
Casey Kasem	Carl Weathers
Cloris Leachman	Dennis Weaver
Paul & Linda McCartney	Paul Winter
Hayley Mills	Gretchen Wyler

This list was compiled from a variety of sources. Carol J. Adams,
The Sexual Politics of Meat; Nathaniel Altman, Eating for Life;

Billy Ray Boyd, For the Vegetarian in You; and EarthSave's Realities for the 90's. This list includes vegetarians, those who eat no meat or fish. They are not necessarily total vegetarians (vegans) who also avoid eggs and dairy products. To read more about well-known vegetarians of the past and present, respectively, see the following books, both written by Rynn Berry: Famous Vegetarians and Their Favorite Recipes (Los Angeles: Panjandrum Books, 1991), and The New Vegetarians (Long Island, NY: Town House Press, 1989).

❄ NOURISHED BY LOVE ❄

1. Choose natural foods from the plant kingdom—*fruits, vegetables, whole grains, and legumes.*

2. These may be eaten generously. *Have ample portions from these four food groups. If you enjoy salad, eat all you want as long as you're not using a rich, oily dressing. (In that case, replace or limit the dressing, not the salad.)*

3. Avoid second helpings as a general rule. *When you serve yourself, start with enough. If someone serves you a piddly portion, have more.*

4. Rethink main course *so that rice, potatoes, or a large salad with pasta or beans in it can fit there. Round out meals with more vegetables, bread, etc.*

5. Use rich relatives like nuts, avocado, and dried fruit sparingly. *(If you're healthy, don't need to lose weight, and can handle extra calories, you can eat more of these.)*

6. Go for quality. *You deserve better than junk food. For the most part, leave sugar, grease, and excess salt on their side of the tracks—the wrong side. Caffeine and alcohol consumption should be reduced or eliminated.*

7. Have three meals a day *unless your doctor wants you to eat more often. Sit down for your meals. Have a place setting. Do your best not to rush.*

8. If you want a snack, have fruit. *Feeling hungry for a while*

before a meal is okay, too. Unless you have a medical condition requiring small, frequent meals, your choosing to go without food between lunch and dinner and between dinner and bedtime will not harm you.

9. Eat only when you're emotionally and spiritually centered. *If you feel you're about to eat for a fix, even at mealtime, get yourself together first by calling a supportive friend, taking a walk, or writing in a journal.*

10. Avoid your personal binge foods, *those that seem to incite overeating or that you obsess over when they're around. The Love-powered diet eliminates most of the common ones, but you need to recognize and respect yours.*

11. Leave a little food on your plate. *I've heard it called the "angel bite." You're not a failure when you don't do this, but you get lots of inner nourishment when you do.*

12. Follow "Nutritional Guidelines" which follows. *Familiarize yourself with the fundamental nutritional information in Chapter 7. Help ensure your general health with the Love-powered life suggestions in Chapter 9.*

13. Give less power to the scale. *Find a sensible midpoint between frequent weighing and refusing to find out what you weigh. Decide on once or twice a month and stay with that. You will lose weight. Give yourself an edge with exercise.*[20]

14. Get the help you need. *Continue to ask God or your Higher Self each morning for help in eating reasonably that day. Say thanks at night, even if your eating wasn't perfect. Attend OA. Read the books in Appendix A.*

15. Give yourself priority status. *Allow yourself time for meals and food preparation, for meditation, exercise, support group*

---

20. If you have a history of crash dieting, or if you have been bulimic, it may take time for your body to respond to normal, healthful eating with the loss of weight you're looking for. Be patient. Concentrate on self-acceptance and on enjoying the day at hand. Remember that you're working with the laws of nature. They can't be rushed and they can't be cheated. Allow yourself to be a part of the natural process. This is for life, so there's *no reason to hurry.* Don't be discouraged by a slow-moving scale. If you want to be impressed by a number, look at your Love-powered cholesterol level!

meetings, and whatever else you need. This isn't selfishness, it's self-preservation.

◄ NUTRITIONAL GUIDELINES ►

The love-powered diet provides optimum nutrition for your health. Following these guidelines will further ensure that. If you are under a doctor's care, consult him or her about your eating plan.

If you are pregnant or nursing, follow the advice of your health care provider. For additional information, see Pregnancy, Children & the Vegan Diet by Michael Klaper, M.D. (available from The American Vegan Society, Appendix C) or The Vegan Diet During Pregnancy, Lactation, and Childhood by Reed Mangels, Ph.D., R.D. (from The Vegetarian Reosurce Group, Appendix C).

1. *Eat from all four Love-powered food groups daily: vegetables, fruits, whole grains, and legumes.*

2. *Have at least one large salad every day and include in it a variety of leafy greens (romaine, leaf lettuce, spinach, etc.) plus other vegetables.*

3. *Include foods rich in vitamin C such as citrus fruits, cantaloupe, bell peppers, tomatoes, and strawberries.*

4. *Eating foods with a high vitamin C content along with iron-rich foods helps increase iron absorption by your body. High iron foods include dried beans, peas, and lentils, dried fruit such as prunes and figs, almonds, cashews, whole grains, and leafy greens (the greens come with their own vitamin C as well).*

5. *Include at least two daily servings of calcium rich foods— collards, kale, broccoli, oatmeal, soybeans, tofu cultured with calcium sulfate, calcium-fortified orange juice, almonds. (Virtually all your food will provide some calcium, and much research indicates that people need less of this mineral on a plant-based diet than on one high in animal protein. See Chapter 7.)*

6. *Be sure to get moderate exposure to sunlight during good weather for vitamin D. This is of particular concern to dark-skinned people living in northern latitudes.*

7. *If you have used no animal products for three years, or if you are pregnant or nursing, supplement your diet regularly with a source of vitamin B$_{12}$ (cobalamin) to meet the RDA of 2 micrograms daily. B$_{12}$ tablets contain more than this and may be taken weekly. Many vegetarian foods are fortified with B$_{12}$, including some meat analogs, nutritional yeasts, powdered soy milks, and some commonly available cereals, such as Nutri-Grain and Kellogg's Bran Flakes. (For more on vitamin B$_{12}$, consult Chapter 7.)*

8. *Eat a vegetable from the cabbage family (broccoli, brussels sprouts, cauliflower, etc.) at least four times a week.*

9. *The Love-powered diet will keep your protein intake at the proper level. Provided you obtain adequate calories from a variety of natural foods, you will secure ample protein without special foods or food combinations. Don't overdo protein by eating too many beans—a cup a day is plenty.*

10. *To keep fat consumption low, be moderate in your use of nuts, seeds, olives, and avocado, and be ever so sparing in your use of oil for cooking and salad dressings. Cut down by water-sautéing, substituting applesauce for shortening in baking, and using nonstick cookware. (See "Fat Zappers" in Chapter 8.) However, note "the vegan factor," as Michael Klaper, M.D., explains, "This means a person eating in the vegan style eats NO animal fats, and thus normally consumes a very lowfat diet, free of cholesterol and many of the saturated fats inherent in animal products. . . . Consequently, the modest use of olive and safflower oil for recipes, and minimal amounts of (heat stable) coconut oil for quick frying, is approved. . . . With any oil, however, use the smallest amount possible; just brushing the bottom of the pan with a light coating, rather than pouring in a large volume of oil, will leave the food and the palate less greasy."[21]*

21. Michael Klaper, M. D., *Vegan Nutrition: Pure and Simple*, p. 45. (See Appendix A.)

—❦—

SEVEN

Healthy

and Whole

This is a technology alert. By that I mean that the upcoming chapter is fairly detailed in its discussion of nutrition and health as they relate to a Love-powered diet. This important information can help you confidently make this change in your eating habits, plan meals that will best support your health, and answer the questions you're sure to be asked when people see that you are eating differently. You may want to share this chapter with your doctor or nutritionist, but if you're not up for figures, facts, and footnotes right now, feel free to skip ahead and come back to this later.

People are very trusting about nutrition. Oh, we can sound pretty sophisticated talking about amino acids and polyunsaturates. Even so, don't you think most people believe that anything on a grocer's shelf (that doesn't have a skull and crossbones on it) is, if not a full-fledged health food, at least quite suitable for human consumption? Most folks pride themselves on being omnivorous. "I can eat any-thing" and "I have a cast-iron stomach" are boastful statements. Nevertheless, the *results* of eating everything edible and treating our stomachs as if they were indeed formed in a smelter, are devastating.

We see these results in overweight, digestive disorders, and de-generative disease. What's more, this seems normal. Repeated diets, popping antacids, even submitting to major surgery are practices so common they're regarded as inevitable. The Love-powered diet, although not a panacea, may be an alternative. When introduced to it, however, people often respond defensively. They want to know, "Where do you get your protein? Where do you get your cal-cium? Where do you get your iron?" The answer is that all these nutrients come to us from the plant kingdom. By eating plant foods, we get them directly. With animal foods, we get them second hand.

Still, most people eat everything and assume that doing so is essen-tial for good health. That assumption has been substantiated over the years with the assorted caveats applied to vegetarian diets. These in-clude such assertions as:

* It's all right not to eat meat, but you need to have plenty of milk and eggs, and maybe some fish every so often.

* Vegetarians need to take lots of supplements—protein powder and bone meal and cod liver oil.

* Well, you *can* eat that way if you combine your food just so and plan every meal very, very carefully.

I'll bet skydivers and hang glider pilots don't get such persistent warnings! Amazingly, not one of these has an actual basis in current scientific information. On the contrary, "It's easier to balance a vege-tarian diet," writes William Harris, M.D. "You can tie yourself in knots juggling calories, nutrients, and cholesterol on an omnivorous diet. Plant foods are nutrient-dense and modest in calories with zero cholesterol, so the diet takes care of itself."[1]

Isn't that too easy? No, it's just easy enough. And it's one important reason why this eating style can be a helpful tool for keeping food obsession from resurfacing: you don't have to spend an inordinate amount of time thinking about your food. Natural, vegetarian meals are complete and nourishing. Your body knows what to do with them so you can stop counting, quantifying, measuring, and worrying about what you eat. You can put your mind on other things.

The purpose of this chapter is to provide you with fundamental information. The approach we'll take for doing that will be to first look at some of the problems of the Standard American Diet (we can call it SAD) and how eating the Love-powered way can help solve them. Then we'll consider specific health problems common in the western world and how this kind of food has been shown effective in preventing and even reversing many of these. Finally, we will consider the relative merits of Love-powered eating and the traditional Four Food Groups approach, and discuss the specific nutrients would-be vegetarians are often concerned about.

◀ WHAT'S SO SAD ABOUT THE ▶ THE STANDARD AMERICAN DIET?

The prestigious journals of medicine and nutrition have for decades been dotted with reports connecting the way people eat with many of the ills they endure. A great many of these studies show that vegetarian or near-vegetarian diets can reduce the risk for many of the diseases and disorders that plague modern society. Apparently, several key differences exist between a natural, vegetarian diet (the Love-powered diet) and the Standard American Diet (SAD). The Love-powered diet is based on vegetable foods; it's low in fat, high in fiber, and moderate in protein. The SAD, on the other hand, is built around animal foods, is high in fat, deficient in fiber, and excessive in protein. Let's examine each of these differences.

---

1. From "Going Vegetarian" by William Harris, M.D., in *Guide to Healthy Eating*, Physicians Committee for Responsible Medicine, March–April 1989.

Animal Foods

Michael Klaper, M.D., makes the straightforward declaration, "The body of Homo sapiens has no nutritional requirement for the flesh of animals, for the eggs of chickens, or for the milk of cows."[2] Not only can we be well-nourished without them, there is ample evidence that such foods are actually harmful. In addition to the overload of cholesterol, fat, and protein in most of them and their dearth of fiber (these will be discussed shortly), animal foods are also the major dietary source of purines which cause a rise in fat and glucose levels in the blood, a rise likely to encourage fat storage in the body.[3] Meats are deficient in carbohydrate, the food component that should account for sixty to eighty percent of the calories ingested. (Carbohydrate-deficient diets lead to decreased endurance.) Stress hormones secreted by the animal prior to slaughter also become a part of the meat.[4] In addition, chemical contaminants concentrate in the tissues of animals, and these contaminants are taken in by those who consume the animal's meat and milk. Joseph Weissman, M.D., explains:

> All animals, including humans, are bioconcentrators and biomagnifiers. Pesticides and other poisonous chemicals do enter the food chain from the soil to [grasses], fruits and vegetables, but in most cases the toxins absorbed by plants remain at the same level of concentration as the original soil. However, animals concentrate and store the poisons they eat. Many of these toxins are fat-soluble and make their home in the fatty and cholesterol areas of the host animal.

Because the levels of toxins in animal foods are much higher than those in plants (by a factor of sixteen in some studies), eating plants

2. Michael Klaper, M.D., *Vegan Nutrition: Pure and Simple*, "Foreword for Health Professionals." (See Appendix A.)
3. Agatha Thrash, M.D., and Calvin Thrash, M.D., *Nutrition for Vegetarians* (Seale, AL: New Lifestyles Books, 1982), p. 119. This ability of purines to elevate blood levels of fat and glucose also applies to the caffeine in coffee, black and maté teas, cola drinks and some medications, and to the theobromine found in cocoa.
4. "Just before and during the agony of being slaughtered, large quantities of adrenaline are forced through the entire body, thus 'pain poisoning' the entire carcass. Even the meat industry acknowledges that preslaughter psychological stress produces physical changes in the carcass." Nathaniel Altman, *Eating for Life* (NY: Vegetus, 1986), p. 72.

instead of animals greatly reduces our intake of these poisons.[5] Of course, choosing organic produce can also result in a marked decrease in the amount of synthetic pesticides that we consume. Even so, it is believed that the average person consumes far more of these in animal than in vegetable foods.

And pesticide residues aren't the only extras in a slab of steak or bucket of chicken. Growth hormones are commonly used in livestock production, and fifty-five percent of the antibiotics used in the U.S. are routinely fed to animals on farms. Although this practice is banned by the entire European Economic Community, it is deemed necessary in this country to keep animals reared in factory farm confinement well and growing. It is also, however, believed to have contributed to the marked rise in antibiotic-resistant infections over the past thirty years.[6]

Fish, too, although not intentionally fed potential toxins by humans, are subject to the effects of chemical runoff in our rivers, lakes, and seas. Many fish show serious concentrations of heavy metals, mutation-inducing hydrocarbons, and radioactivity from nuclear pollution. They also exhibit an alarming incidence of cancer.[7]

High in Fat

The typical Western diet with its reliance on meats, fish, eggs, and dairy products, along with fried foods and rich baked goods, provides too much fat—forty percent of calories on average—as well as artery-clogging cholesterol. Fats carry calories at more than double the amount of either proteins or carbohydrates.[8] In other words, eating fat means getting more calories from less food. Eating enough high-fat

5. Joseph D. Weissman, M.D., *Choose to Live* (New York: Grove Press, 1988), pp. 26–27.
6. Irvin Moltolsky, "Animal Antibiotics Tied to Illnesses in Humans," *New York Times*, February, 22, 1987, cited in *Realities for the 90's*, the EarthSave booklet citing facts from *Diet for a New America* by John Robbins.
7. For details see *Vegan Nutrition: Pure and Simple* by Michael Klaper, M.D., pp. 18–20.
8. Fat contains 9 calories per gram. Protein contains 4 calories per gram, as does carbohydrate as sugar. Starch, a combination of carbohydrate, fiber, and water, has 1 calorie per gram. (John McDougall, M.D., *The McDougall Plan*, p. 123.)

foods to feel full is likely to lead to weight gain, but cutting portion sizes to include these foods results in leaving the table hungry—the first step in the demise of one more diet.

Not only do fats have more calories than other foods, the body likes to hang on to calories from fat. It's a physiological principle that many of the excess calories from carbohydrates are stored in the liver as glycogen so they can be drawn on for use as energy. According to John McDougall, M.D., fats ingested in foods can be appropriated for body fat much more easily.[9]

Animal foods have, as a rule, a much higher fat content than do vegetables, fruits, grains, and legumes. In addition, animal fats are of a different type than vegetable fats. They are primarily saturated,[10] and it is saturated fat that plays a part in elevating blood cholesterol levels.

Cholesterol itself is made in the livers of animals, including humans. We make all we need. The cholesterol obtained from food is extra and accounts in part for the abnormally high blood cholesterol levels prevalent in this country. As pointed out earlier in this book, dietary cholesterol is found exclusively in animal foods, so eating the Love-powered way means taking in none of it. Why is this a good idea? While numerous studies have associated elevated cholesterol levels with heart disease, a low blood cholesterol level may be a reasonable indicator of protection against other degenerative conditions as well. Early findings from the "Cornell-China-Oxford Project on Nutrition, Health and Environment"[11] indicate:

> The higher the plasma cholesterol level, the higher is the risk for so-called diseases of affluence—cancers, heart disease, diabetes, the kinds

9. From a lecture by John McDougall, M.D., American Vegan Society conference, Arcata, CA, Aug. 1989.
10. A few plant foods—primarily coconut, chocolate, and palm oil—are also high in saturated fat.
11. This study, a monumental joint venture of American, British, and Chinese researchers, is an unusually comprehensive study of diet and health. It looked at the eating habits of 6,500 Chinese people. The study is unique not only in its vastness but because of its locale: In China, people generally live in the same area all their lives and eat the foods native to that region. Diseases tend to occur there in regional clusters, making for an unparalleled research opportunity. It will take many years for all the data obtained to be interpreted, but initial findings clearly indicate that a vegetarian or at least a near-vegetarian diet is optimal for prevention of degenerative disease.

of disease we see in the West. This is pretty remarkable because the plasma cholesterols in China are between about 100 and 200 milligrams per deciliter. In other words, their high is our low. What it's really saying in a sense is the lower the cholesterol level the better. High cholesterol levels are related to the consumption of animal foods—and it apparently doesn't take very much of them.[12]

Even the so-called lean cuts of meat have significant levels of saturated fat plus cholesterol. Eating poultry is only a slight improvement and even fish can be extremely high in cholesterol, even though most fish is lower in fat content than meat. There are some vegetable foods which are high in fat (the rich relatives introduced in Chapter 6—oils, margarine, nuts, seeds, olives, avocado and, to a lesser degree, soybean products), but the fat in these foods is primarily unsaturated. These fats have not been implicated in heart disease as have the saturated fats prevalent in animal foods, but it's wise to avoid an excess of all fats. Some studies have shown that high quantities of vegetable oils can exacerbate the growth of tumors, and both saturated and unsaturated fats have the same (high) caloric density.

Love-powered eating outshines the Standard American Diet in that the latter gives high-fat foods such as meat and eggs star billing at meals. Milk, eggs, butter, and cheese are also used in preparing other foods from side dishes to desserts, and high-fat vegetable foods— salad and cooking oil, margarine, peanut butter—are used as well. The Love-powered diet eliminates cholesterol and most saturated fat, so the majority of people can enjoy moderate use of the richer plant foods without difficulty.

Deficient in Fiber

Meat and dairy products are devoid of the plant fiber required for normal peristaltic action of the colon. In addition, the refining of grains removes most of their fiber content. The upshot of all this is that difficulties of digestion and elimination are so common in "well-fed" so-

12. T. Colin Campbell, Ph.D., Cornell University nutritional biochemist who was the key American researcher in the project. Telephone interview with author, February, 1991.

cieties that bran flakes, fiber-enriched breads, and natural fiber laxatives are common as well. Actually, fiber shouldn't have to be added *to* the diet. It ought to be *in* the diet already.

"The only reason you have a laxative industry is because you've taken the fiber out of your diet," cancer researcher and authority on fiber, Denis Burkitt, M.D., told Dr. Neal Barnard for his book *The Power of Your Plate*.[13] High-fiber diets help lower cholesterol by trapping bile acids in the intestinal tract and allowing them to be excreted, and such a diet is believed to protect against varicose veins, hemorrhoids, hiatus hernia, appendicitis, and gallstones, as well as constipation.[14]

The richest sources of fiber are whole grains and legumes, and vegetables and fruits are fiber-filled as well. If you recognize these as the Love-powered foursome, you're exactly right!

Excessive in Protein

Not long ago, high protein was a sort of buzzword for good nutrition, but we were misled on that one. Protein is certainly necessary, but most people get far too much of it and that can be a serious problem. No more than fifteen percent of calories in a normal diet should come from protein, but Americans routinely eat animal foods that contain forty-one percent (skim milk, turkey), seventy-nine percent (cottage cheese), even eighty-eight percent (water-packed tuna).[15]

Although you may have heard that protein burns fat, this assertion is based on the disease state of ketosis that occurs when you consume a risky diet of virtually only protein and fat, no carbohydrate. In actuality, it is more likely that a high intake of protein—especially that from animal sources—may lead to overweight. In the China health study cited earlier, it was learned that the Chinese consume, on average, twenty percent more calories per pound of body weight than do

13. Denis Burkitt, M.D., quoted by Neal Barnard, M.D., in *The Power of Your Plate*, p. 121. (See Appendix A.)
14. Neal Barnard, M.D., *The Power of Your Plate*, pp. 121–25.
15. John McDougall, M.D., *The McDougall Plan*, p. 105. Note that these very high protein foods are also among those animal foods lowest in fat and therefore often used to replace their higher fat but lower protein counterparts. This is not a fully profitable trade-off. Reducing the fat in dairy foods, for example, causes a rise in their per calorie protein. Excess protein in the diet can cause problems just as excess fat can.

Americans, but the Chinese are lighter and leaner than we are by some twenty-five percent. Part of the reason for this is likely to be their somewhat higher amount of physical exercise. The Chinese diet is also one that is low in fat. But Cornell researcher T. Colin Campbell believes that protein intake, animal protein in particular, may play a part as well:

> It turns out that when one is on a low intake of animal protein, a higher proportion of the energy consumed is actually burned off as heat and it is not laid down as body fat. So a low-protein diet, which is characteristic of a vegetarian type of diet, allows obviously more energy to be consumed without running into the risk of getting fat from that extra energy, those extra calories. This is an old observation incidentally. It's been around many, many years, although it's been really much ignored. It's clear that if you look at vegans in this country, they tend to be rather lean. They tend not to have obesity problems."[16]

John Scharffenberg, M.D., of Loma Linda University, has listed other problems with excess protein in the diet, beginning with the fact that it "increases excretion of calcium—tending to cause a loss of bone mass (osteoporosis)—increases the work of the liver and kidneys, and shortens life span.

"Surprisingly, high protein intake can also result in excessive vitamin losses. For example, because protein mobilizes vitamin A from the liver into the bloodstream, high protein intake increases the requirement for vitamin A."[17] (Ironically, one of the symptoms of true protein deficiency is inability to absorb vitamin A from the intestine. In other words, we need enough, not more than enough.)

Disease Prevention—The Vegetarian Edge

If I tell you that the proof of all this is in the pudding, you could tell me I'm using a food addict's favorite phrase, but there is absolute truth in it. Among the ways in which vegetarians are generally better off than omnivores are:

16. T. Colin Campbell, Ph.D., telephone interview with author, February, 1991.
17. John A. Scharffenberg, M.D., *Problems With Meat*. (Santa Barbara: Woodbridge Press Publ. Co., 1979, 1982), p. 82. (Dr. Scharffenberg footnotes all these assertions with references to the medical literature.)

Obesity. Vegetarians who consume milk and eggs tend to be slightly leaner than average, but vegans (total vegetarians—people whose diet resembles the Love-powered diet) are almost always so.

Heart Disease. Vegans have very low cholesterol levels and a concurrently low incidence of heart disease. This finding is not new. Back in June of 1961, an editorial in the *Journal of the American Medical Association* stated that a total vegetarian diet "could prevent 90% of our thromboembolic disease and 97% of our coronary occlusions."[18] It was only in the late 1980s, however, that the work of Dean Ornish, M.D., and his colleagues at the University of California at San Francisco, confirmed that coronary artery disease can be not only prevented but *reversed* with a lowfat, vegetarian diet in combination with lifestyle modification including exercise and stress management techniques.[19]

Blood Pressure. Studies repeatedly show that a lowfat vegetarian diet tends to produce lower blood pressure. This could be due to the trimness of vegetarians, but they also show markedly lower blood viscosity (thickness). The hormonal factors present in meat may also play a role. George Eisman, R.D., explains: "Stress hormones are present in an animal at the time of slaughter. The same hormones that cause animals' blood pressure to rise cause ours to rise. It just takes a few molecules."[20]

Diabetes. The decreased chance of obesity in total vegetarians puts them at lower risk for developing adult-onset diabetes. In addition, "A high-fat diet, even if it doesn't lead to obesity, may bring on diabetes in genetically predisposed individuals—perhaps because the cells of the body are so clogged with fat that they don't receive the insulin message to remove sugar from the bloodstream. The sugar (glucose) accumulates in the blood with disastrous results." Lowfat diets high in unrefined carbohydrates have clinical application in treating diabetes.[21] Administered under a physician's care, such diets frequently

---

18. Editorial, "Diet and Stress in Vascular Disease," *Journal of the American Medical Association* 176(9) (1961): 806–7.
19. For more on this, see *Dr. Dean Ornish's Program for Reversing Heart Disease.*
20. George Eisman, M.S., R.D., telephone interview with author, March, 1991.
21. Among the physicians taking this approach is Julian M. Whitaker, M.D. His book on the subject is *Reversing Diabetes* (New York: Warner Books, 1987).

result in elimination of medication (insulin or oral hypoglycemic agents) in adult-onset diabetics and reduction in insulin, as well as better general control, for those with juvenile diabetes.

Osteoporosis. The brittle bone disease that primarily affects post-menopausal women is less likely to occur among vegetarians because they do not have the high intake of protein that causes calcium to be leached from the bones. Adequate but modest protein consumption combined with regular, weight-bearing exercise, appears to be the best defense against osteoporosis. Supplementary calcium has not been conclusively proven effective, and when extra calcium is taken in the form of dairy products, any possible benefit from the calcium may be offset by the additional protein ingested in the milk or cheese. (See "Calcium or Cowcium?" later in this chapter.)

Breast Cancer. Women who eat meat daily (compared to those who eat it less than once a week) increase their risk of developing breast cancer 3.8 times. Those who eat eggs daily (compared to once a week) increase their risk of breast cancer 2.8 times.[22] Factors accounting for this may include the way vegetarian women process estrogen, retaining less of it in their bodies than do meat-eaters, and the later onset of menses in the females of more vegetarian populations. (Early puberty appears to be related to increased incidence of breast cancer. "Age of menarche is markedly delayed among young Chinese women, ranging from 15.2 to 18.9 years. Mean menarchal age in the U.S. is around 12 years. . . . Diets rich in energy, protein, calcium, fat and other growth-stimulating factors, when consumed by the sexually immature youth, enhance the rate of growth, causing earlier onset of menarche."[23])

Other Diseases. Some other cancers, including those of the ovaries, prostate, colon, and rectum, are statistically less common among vegetarians. Eliminating or drastically reducing meat consumption is standard in the treatment of gout (the purines in meat seem to be the

---

22. These figures come from a paper presented by Takeshi Hirayama at the Conference on Breast Cancer and Diet, US-Japan Cooperative Cancer Research Program, Seattle, March, 1977. Cited in the EarthSave booklet *Realities for the 90's.*
23. T. Colin Campbell, Ph.D., "The Study on Diet, Nutrition and Disease in the People's Republic of China," *Contemporary Nutrition* 14:6, 1989.

aggravating factor here) and kidney failure (in this case, intake of all high-protein foods is curtailed). Studies have shown vegetarians to have a decreased incidence of gallstones, kidney stones, diverticular disease, and stroke. Stroke is the obstruction of an artery to the brain. When an artery to the heart is completely blocked, heart attack occurs. The same condition—saturated fat and cholesterol impeding blood flow—can account for either. It's merely a matter of location.

In fact, this type of blockage (atherosclerosis) has been implicated in impotence in males. "A study of 440 impotent men was published in the *Lancet* in January, 1985. The same risk factors that have been identified for heart disease were present in the impotent men to a greater extent than in the general population. Just as in heart disease, a disruption of blood flow leads to a loss of function. The study concluded that the increase in the frequency of impotence with age is mainly related to atherosclerosis."[24]

This information should tell us that switching to a Love-powered diet is the smartest move to take in terms of eating habits to provide the best odds for a long, healthy, enjoyable life. It would make sense that the same food program that protects against so many diseases and lacks so many of the components shown to be harmful to human health would also provide us with what we need nutritionally. "Nutshell Nutrition," at the end of this chapter, provides a brief overview of nutritional basics. At this point, let's examine in some detail how the Love-powered diet rates against the Four Food Groups most of us grew up with. At first glance, a Love-powered diet made up primarily of whole grains, legumes, vegetables, and fruits seems to be woefully inadequate in light of the Basic Four's meat, dairy, fruit/vegetable, and bread/cereal groups. In eliminating meats and dairy products, a Love-powered diet appears to deprive anyone who eats it of fully half the foods needed for health. How can this be?

---

24. Neal D. Barnard, M.D., "Diet and Sexual Potency," *The Animals' Agenda*, June 1990, citing the work of R. Virag, P. Bouilly, and D. Frydman, "Is impotence an arterial disorder? A study of arterial risk factors in 440 impotent men." *Lancet* 1:181–84, 1985.

◀ THE MYTH OF THE FOUR FOOD GROUPS ▶

Contrary to the belief of many, the Four Food Groups were not a foot-note to the Ten Commandments. The system was instead devised in 1956 by the United States Department of Agriculture (USDA) as a simplification of the earlier Basic Seven, developed during World War II to streamline the unwieldy Basic Twelve formulated in the 1930s. That earliest listing read:

1. Milk and milk products
2. Potatoes and sweet potatoes
3. Dry mature peas, beans, and nuts
4. Tomatoes and citrus fruits
5. Leafy green and yellow vegetables
6. Other vegetables and fruits
7. Eggs
8. Lean meat, poultry, and fish
9. Flour and cereals
10. Butter
11. Other fats
12. Sugars.[25]

The Basic Seven condensed these to:

1. Meat, poultry, fish, eggs, dried beans and peas, nuts
2. Leafy green and yellow vegetables
3. Citrus fruits, raw cabbage, salad greens, and tomatoes
4. Other vegetables and noncitrus fruits
5. Bread, breakfast cereals, and flour
6. Butter and fortified margarine
7. Milk and milk products.[26]

25. This list is from research by Nathaniel Altman for his article, "Nutritional Water-gate: The Story of the 'Four Food Groups,'" parts of which were published in several magazines in the late 1970s. Altman provided research material and assistance for this section of Chapter 7.
26. *World Book Encyclopedia*, vol. 14, p. 632, 1990.

Three major changes took place when the cut from seven to four was made. First, the fruits and vegetables which had comprised three groups were compressed into one, raising the percentage of animal food groups (meat, eggs, and dairy) recommended from twenty-eight and one-half to fifty percent! Secondly, since the Basic Seven included the Meat Group in a listing of concentrated protein foods including pulses and nuts, that percentage leap favoring animal foods was actually greater than the numbers show. Please note than none of this reflected any change in human nutritional needs but was instead a mere categorical substitution. Recently the Meat Group has begun to be referred to as the Meat and Meat Substitute Group, an improvement in nomenclature but still implying that nonmeat protein sources are only substitutes for the real thing.

Finally, the Four Food Groups, unlike the Basic Seven and its predecessor, have no listing for fats and oils. The Four Food Groups allow for a high fat intake in the form of meat, eggs, and dairy, but in failing to acknowledge other fats and oils, the Basic Four may unwittingly foster the idea that they don't count, that eating from the listed groups is sufficient for good nutrition regardless of what is consumed in addition to that.

Still, people *believe* in the Basic Four and are often surprised to learn that it is not universally accepted. Canada, for example, has five groups, giving fruits and vegetables each a category. The Food and Nutrition Center in the Philippines recommends six food groups:

1. Leafy and yellow vegetables
2. Vitamin C-rich foods, including papaya, citrus, melons, and tomatoes
3. Other fruits, including pineapple, jackfruit, okra, and avocado
4. Fat-rich foods, including butter and margarine, coconut milk, and oil
5. Protein-rich foods, such as milk, fish, poultry, red meat, eggs, dried beans and nuts
6. Rice and other energy foods, including bread and root vegetables.[27]

27. This information was quoted by Nathaniel Altman from *Foundations of Nutrition*, 6th ed., by Taylor and Pye (Macmillan, New York, 1966), p. 50.

Different foods are, of course, eaten in different cultures and there is the temptation to see various nations' dietary recommendations as a nutritional version of "to each his own." However, physiologically we are one species and as discussed at length earlier on, some foods can, when used frequently, contribute to chronic disease. Eating the recommended amounts from the traditional Four Food Groups (two or more servings from the meat group, three or more from the milk group, and four or more from each of the fruit/vegetable and bread/cereal groups[28]) can ensure acquisition of the nutritional elements sufficient to prevent deficiency diseases. However,

> The Basic Four plan provides merely a minimum guide to nutrients; it sets no limit on calories, saturated fats, cholesterol or protein (which, we have now learned, is as dangerous in excess as it is in deficiency). . . . Because two out of the four groups are animal derived—generally rich in one or more of these food components—fingers have been pointed at the Basic Four Food Groups as a promoter of these excesses.

> The Basic Four plan also fails to recognize the importance of fiber. . . . For example, the Basic Four's Bread and Cereal Group now recommends using "enriched or whole grain products," thereby putting milled, fiberless grains on an equal par with their unprocessed, whole-food counterparts. (The original plan did not mention whole grain products *at all*.) Also the Fruit and Vegetable Group does not differentiate between juices, which are basically devoid of fiber, and whole fruits, which are eaten with their fiber content intact.[29]

The death knell may be sounding, however, for the Four Food Groups as we know them. Many respected experts in nutrition and dietetics have pointed out their limitations and are calling for a revised grouping system that more fully reflects the Dietary Guidelines for Americans,[30] which say:

28. George Eisman, M.S., R.D., "Are the Basic Four Valid Today?" *Vegetarian Times*, October 1987, p. 16.
29. Eisman, as above, p. 18.
30. The Dietary Guidelines for Americans came about as a joint venture of the U.S. Department of Agriculture and the U.S. Department of Health and Human Services. Among the scientific bases for the Guidelines were *The Surgeon General's Report on Nutrition and Health*, 1988, from the Public Health Service, U.S. Department of Health and Human Services; *Diet and Health: Implications for Reducing Chronic Disease*,

- Eat a variety of foods
- Maintain a healthy weight
- Choose a diet low in fat, saturated fat, and cholesterol
- Choose a diet with plenty of vegetables, fruits, and grain products
- Use sugars only in moderation
- Use salt and sodium only in moderation
- If you drink alcoholic beverages, do so in moderation

In the spring of 1991, the USDA was prepared to present a revised version of food groups based on the Dietary Guidelines for Americans. The revision was to illustrate food families as a pyramid, with grains as its broad base, implying that these should form the bulk of a healthful diet. Next on the pyramid were fruits and vegetables, shown as separate groups. As the pyramid narrowed, it included dairy products and a protein group including animal and vegetable sources of concentrated protein. The tip was for fats and sweets to be used sparingly.

Knowing what you do now, you can see that this represented quite an improvement. Nevertheless, the pyramid design was never officially released because it was seen as being too complicated. Some observers at the time noted that industry pressure rather than graphic complexity was the real reason that, for now anyway, the Four Food Groups have yet to be usurped.

With coincidental timing, just before the USDA was to have introduced its Eating Right Pyramid, an independent organization, Physicians Committee for Responsible Medicine (see Appendix C), unveiled its own plan, The New Four Food Groups, at a Washington, D.C., news conference. Presenting these were T. Colin Campbell, Ph.D., professor of nutritional biochemistry at Cornell University and director of the Chinese health study noted earlier; Denis Burkitt, M.D., an acclaimed physician and expert on dietary fiber; Oliver Alabaster, M.D., director of the Institute for Disease Prevention at the George Washington University Medical Center; and Neal Barnard,

and *Recommended Daily Allowances*, 10th ed., both 1989 publications of the National Research Council, National Academy of Sciences. The Guidelines are quoted from Home and Garden Bulletin No. 232, from the USDA and the U.S. Department of Health & Human Services.

M.D., associate director of Behavioral Studies in the Institute for Disease Prevention at George Washington University and president of Physicians Committee for Responsible Medicine.

What did these luminaries come up with as The New Four Food Groups? The same things as you and I when back in Chapter 6, we decided that a Love-powered diet was comprised of vegetables, fruits, whole grains, and legumes. PCRM's explanation of these is given on page 143, along with suggested numbers of daily servings for each group. This grouping does not carry a governmental seal of approval, but it stands up under scientific scrutiny *and* it can make for very good eating. If you have any doubts about the latter, see page 145, the menu served at the press conference when The New Four Food Groups made their debut.

It is gratifying to see knowledgeable professionals formulate nutritional guidelines that are ideal for both human and planetary health. Even without a system of food groups, however, it is not difficult to plan an adequate diet from natural, vegetarian foods. Nature has designed these to meet our needs not just adequately but abundantly. Of course some planning is required, particularly because lowfat, vegetarian foods are not yet the major menu items at the fast-food restaurants and roadside diners which often seem to be the most convenient places to stop for a meal. Your choice of restaurants will gradually change as your style of eating changes, and you may find that you like your own cooking more and more.

Both cooking and eating out will be explored in depth in the upcoming chapter, but for now we'll finish up on nutrition by looking at the specific nutrients many people fear they could miss when they make the transition to Love-powered eating. These are protein, iron, calcium, riboflavin, and vitamin B_{12}.[31]

Protein Again

We've talked about getting too much. At this point, let's talk about getting enough. If you could design a diet built around natural starches and vegetables that provided enough calories to maintain

---

31. Questions are also sometimes asked about vitamin D and zinc. See pages 150 and 152 for information on these as well as on other vitamins and minerals.

normal weight but was deficient in protein, you'd be famous because no one has been able to do so yet. The only way a person on a natural foods, animal-free diet could become deficient in protein would be to take in too few calories due to excessive fasting or dieting, anorexia, or famine; or to live solely on those few fruits or other natural foods that are quite low in protein (less than five percent of calories).

But what about amino acids, those building blocks of protein that some believe vegetarians could only obtain by eating grains, legumes, and nuts in precise mathematical combinations? You can save your calculator for doing your taxes. You won't need it to prepare your dinner. Eat a variety of natural foods over the course of the day and protein complementing will take care of itself. "In fact," says George Eisman, R.D., "all plant proteins are complete. Some are higher in certain amino acids than others, but by eating enough of any one plant protein, all needs can be adequately met. The irony is that an incomplete protein *does* exist: it's gelatin, an animal derivative."[32]

Page 147 shows a protein summary. Also, books recommended in Appendix A that deal with nutrition can provide more details.

The Popeye Principle

Natural vegetarian foods make a respectable showing in terms of iron content and some of them—such as dried fruits (prunes, dried apricots, raisins, dried peaches), dried beans and lentils, whole grains such as rye and wheat, as well as green, leafy vegetables—are all rich in this mineral. However, it has long been held that iron from animal sources (heme iron) is more readily assimilated than nonheme iron from plants. Also, phytates present in whole grains have been believed to detrimentally inhibit iron utilization, although this has never been known to cause iron deficiency in a human. Suzanne Havala, R.D., has done research into the iron sufficiency of vegetarian diets, based in large part on the Chinese study mentioned earlier. She says:

In research, the focus is often on single or isolated nutrients or other substances. Results often ignore the reality of the complexity of nu-

32. George Eisman, M.S., R.D., telephone interview with author, March, 1991.

trient interactions that occur within the context of the total diet. In this case, plant components such as fiber and phytates apparently do not have a significant effect on iron absorption in vegetarian diets that contain adequate vitamin C from fruits and vegetables. Vegetarians in the United States tend to have good iron status.[33]

The Chinese have a mean iron intake almost double that of Americans, and although nearly all of this comes from plant foods, "iron status among Chinese adults appears to be adequate with virtually no evidence of anemia, though anemia among children and pregnant mothers was not measured."[34] Iron deficiency anemia is not uncommon in the United States, particularly among women of childbearing age who lose iron during menstruation. Restrictive diets for weight control can be a cause of low iron status, but so can excessive consumption of milk and cheese. Dairy foods are not only deficient in iron; they are antagonistic by actually inhibiting iron utilization.

Dairy products are the cause of at least 50 percent of childhood iron deficiency anemia and an unknown percentage of anemia found in adults; this condition results from bleeding of the small intestine caused by dairy proteins and is not responsive to iron therapy until milk and other dairy foods are eliminated.[35]

Just as iron absorption can be impeded, it can also be enhanced. One way to do this is to eat one or more foods rich in vitamin C (citrus, tomatoes, bell pepper) along with an iron-rich food. Another way to add iron to the diet is to use cast-iron cookware. "It was found that a 100-gram serving of spaghetti sauce prepared in iron cookware contained 87.5 milligrams of iron compared to only three when cooked in a glass vessel."[36]

(You can find capsulized information on iron and the other nutrients discussed in this chapter on page 149 in "Nutshell Nutrition: The Micronutrients.")

33. Suzanne Havala, R.D., telephone interview with author, February, 1991.
34. T. Colin Campbell, Ph.D., "A Study on Diet, Nutrition and Disease in the People's Republic of China," Contemporary Nutrition, 14:5, 1989.
35. John McDougall, M.D., The McDougall Plan, p. 50.
36. Agatha Thrash, M.D., and Calvin Thrash, M.D., Nutrition for Vegetarians, p. 75, citing C. E. Butterworth, Jr., M.D., "Iron 'Undercontamination?'" Journal of the American Medical Association 220(4):581–82, April 24, 1972.

Calcium or Cowcium?

Perhaps even more ubiquitous than the myth that meat is necessary for protein is the myth that cow's milk is necessary for calcium. This defies logic in several ways. First, over half of the world's population, primarily those of African and Asian descent, lack the enzyme to digest cow's milk. Just because enzyme tablets or liquid can be taken to compensate for this does not make it a disease or abnormality. On the contrary, ability to tolerate dairy foods may in fact be an adaptation to their use rather than an indication of normal digestive capacity. *It is, after all, only the human species that drinks milk after weaning or takes the milk of another animal.* All the calcium in cow's milk comes from the grass and grain eaten by the cow. We, too, can get all we need from plant foods.

In fact, virtually any vegetable food you might choose has some calcium in it. Dr. Michael Klaper lists as "calcium all-stars" collards, kale, oats, chickpeas (garbanzos), trail mix made of one part almonds to two-thirds part raisins, and calcium-precipitated tofu.[37] (Tofu made with calcium sulfate will say so on the label.) Moreover, the total amount of calcium that you will need on a Love-powered diet is probably lower than you think. This is because the high-protein content of a meat-based diet causes calcium to be withdrawn from the bones. To eliminate the breakdown products of excess protein, the kidneys are forced to work overtime at excreting more urine. Minerals are in that urine, notably calcium.

In researching a magazine article on this subject a few years ago,[38] I spent a week poring over journal articles at the University of Kansas Medical Center Library and was astonished to learn that the countries with the highest consumption of dairy products also have the highest rates of osteoporosis! This is not such an astonishing fact when you realize that those are also nations with high protein intakes. I also

---

37. Michael Klaper, M.D., *Vegan Nutrition: Pure and Simple*, pp. 31, 51.
38. The article, "Breakfast Protein: Why Less Is More" appeared in the April 1989 issue of *American Health* (pp. 131, 132). It included my report on the protein/calcium connection and that of another writer, Susan Lang, on high protein diets' possible role in promoting cancer. Among the research articles I drew from for that work were two from the *American Journal of Clinical Nutrition*: R. Heaney, "Calcium Nutrition and Bone Health in the Elderly," 36:986, 1982, and S. Margen, "Studies in Calcium Metabolism, the Calciuretic Effect of Dietary Protein," 27:584, 1974.

learned during that library stint that studies using human volunteers as subjects had shown that, on a modest protein intake, calcium balance remained positive when only 500 milligrams of calcium were provided and that high protein diets resulted in negative calcium balance when as much as 1,400 milligrams a day of calcium were supplied.

Animal protein may be more of a culprit in this regard than an equal amount of vegetable protein. Work done in the 1980s at the University of Texas Southwestern Medical Center in Dallas showed that human research subjects who were switched from a vegetarian diet to one containing eggs, red meat, poultry, and fish excreted more calcium, although the actual amount of protein ingested remained the same. (The high sulphur content of animal protein is thought to be the cause. In the body, sulphur turns into the acid sulphate which must be buffered; calcium and other minerals are withdrawn from the bones to do this.)

> Although the United States RDA for calcium for [young] adults is 1200 milligrams, this is probably an artifact of the calcium-wasting nature of the high protein, meat-based American style diet. The World Health Organization, with what many feel is a more appropriate view of human nutrition, recommends a more modest protein intake . . . and thus only 500 milligrams of calcium per day. . . . Numerous medical studies have shown that the intake of calcium on a vegan diet is entirely adequate, and that true calcium deficiency on a vegan diet has never been reported.[39]

A Love-powered diet will probably provide less calcium than one containing dairy products, but it will also be free of excess protein and thus help to ensure a positive calcium balance within your body.

Riboflavin

Most Americans get riboflavin (vitamin B$_2$) in dairy products, meat (especially liver), and eggs, so some nutritionists have expressed concern that vegetarians will lack this vitamin. I think that's rather like telling someone who is chauffeured to the office by limousine that

39. Michael Klaper, M.D., *Vegan Nutrition: Pure and Simple*, p. 31.

she's missing something by not driving herself like "most Americans." In fact, riboflavin is found abundantly in leafy greens, legumes, and nutritional yeast, and to a lesser but still significant extent in whole grains. "Deficiency is rare except in gastrointestinal surgery or when the diet is extremely high in refined and concentrated foods, especially the so-called 'empty calorie junk foods.' "[40]

Vitamin B_{12}

Vitamin B_{12} is a fascinating nutrient about which more is probably unknown than known. We do know the following:

- Vitamin B_{12} is an essential nutrient: without it, severe neurological damage can occur
- Only a minuscule amount is needed—the RDA is 2 mcg. per day (those are micrograms—millionths of a gram)
- In almost every case of reported B_{12} deficiency disease, the cause was not a dietary shortfall but the patient's lack of intrinsic factor, a substance produced in the body necessary for the absorption of vitamin B_{12}
- B_{12} is made by microorganisms (bacteria); therefore, it is not known to occur naturally in foods of plant origin that have been scrubbed clean
- It is stored in the body for long periods, three to eight years, but after three years (or immediately in the case of children or pregnant or nursing mothers), total vegetarians need to include in their diets a supplementary source of vitamin B_{12}

Beyond this, there are many unanswered questions. For example, why have those vegans who have not taken supplemental B_{12} fared, almost without exception, so well? One answer is that the tiny amount of B_{12} needed is likely to be "supplied easily by the millions of helpful microbes found in our mouths and intestinal tracts."[41] Also, in cultures less obsessed than ours with cleanliness, people consume bits of

40. Agatha Thrash, M.D., and Calvin Thrash, M.D., *Nutrition for Vegetarians*, pp. 63–64.
41. John McDougall, M.D., *The McDougall Plan*, p. 39, with a reference to M. Albert, "Vitamin B_{12} Synthesis by Human Small Intestinal Bacteria," *Nature* 283 (1980): 781.

dirt with their food—quite likely enough to provide that infinitesimal but essential dose of B_{12}. In countries such as the U.S. with very sanitary conditions, total vegetarians are advised to include a reliable source of biologically available vitamin B_{12} in their diets.

A reliable source can be a supplementary tablet of vitamin B_{12} (cobalamin) to meet the RDA. This usually means taking a tablet about once a week since the requirement for vitamin B_{12} is so small. B_{12} is apparently better absorbed when taken on its own, rather than as part of a multivitamin. The RDA can also be met with regular use of foods fortified with cobalamin, including many of the breakfast cereals at the supermarket. A variety of products sold at natural food stores—some nutritional yeasts, soy milk powders, and mock meats—have been fortified as well. It was formerly believed that some vegetable foods—notably the fermented soy product tempeh—were sources of usable B_{12}. More sophisticated assay techniques have now shown that this is not the case. (Books and articles on nutrition written before 1988 may list vegan foods containing B_{12}.) Therefore, taking a B_{12} supplement or regularly using B_{12} fortified foods is necessary after three years on a total vegetarian diet or immediately if you are pregnant, nursing, or still growing.

One More Thing

A few new vegans actually have to learn how to get enough *calories*. You may be thinking, "I could use more problems like that" but if you do find that you're losing weight too rapidly—anything approaching the rate at which you lost weight on crash diets is too rapid—you may need to increase your portions. The same is true if you're losing weight and don't need to.

You will definitely be eating *more food* by using Love-powered principles than with any other approach you've taken to release weight[42] or maintain the weight that's right for you. **The caloric equivalent of a four-ounce hamburger sandwich and a dozen measly fries is two full cups of brown rice, topped with a cup of cabbage, a cup of**

---

42. Some people find the notion of releasing weight more helpful than thinking in terms of losing weight. What's lost needs to be found; what is released is let go of without an invitation to return.

cauliflower, a cup of mushrooms, and half an onion stir-fried with nearly a tablespoon of olive oil. Since oils are the most calorific foods anywhere, if you decided to steam the vegetables instead, you could *double* their amount or have a wheat roll on the side.

Of course you don't have to be concerned with juggling calories any longer. You'll eat, you'll finish, and then follow your heart to some noble pursuit or great adventure. (Or maybe you'll just wash the dishes, but you won't have to think about food while you're doing it.) Should you need extra calories to maintain normal weight, increase your amounts of the more concentrated foods like bread and pasta, and (unless you have a medical contraindication to this) you can be more liberal in your use of the rich relatives, concentrated sweets like dates and dried fruits and oil-rich foods such as nuts, nutbutters, olives, and avocado.

Vitamin YOU

Foods contain nutrients, but you—your unique physical self and the mind that so influences that body—are a nutrient processor. You are nourished not by what's on your plate, but by what you can assimilate into your body. Nutrient antagonists abound in most modern lives. Excess stress can create a need for more B-complex vitamins; diuretics can deplete potassium supply. A sedentary lifestyle and the use of caffeine, alcohol, cigarettes, birth control pills, certain antibiotics, and even aspirin can drain vitamin and mineral reserves, so it's obvious that your entire way of life affects your nutritional program.

Part of the beauty of the Love-powered way is that it is not primarily about what you eat. The changes in the foods you choose come about as a result of changes in your consciousness, in your awareness, and in your willingness to love yourself and others. When you no longer need to eat for a fix because of a quiet miracle happening to you mentally and spiritually, a Love-powered food style beautifully expresses your inner transformation in an outer sense. Ultimately, the most important nutritional element is *vitamin YOU*. It is activated by contact with a Higher Power, supportive friends, an appreciation of life and every creature that has it, and supplementary doses of gratitude and wonder. With enough vitamin YOU, the rest is just a piece of organically grown apple.

◀▌ THE NEW FOUR FOOD GROUPS[43] ▐▶

Vegetables

Vegetables are packed with nutrients; they provide vitamin C, beta-carotene, riboflavin and other vitamins, iron, calcium, and fiber. Dark green, leafy vegetables such as broccoli, collards, kale, mustard and turnip greens, chicory, or bok choy are especially good sources of these important nutrients. Dark yellow and orange vegetables such as carrots, winter squash, sweet potatoes, and pumpkin provide extra betacarotene. Include generous portions of a variety of vegetables in your diet.

Fruit

Fruits are rich in fiber, vitamin C and betacarotene. Be sure to include at least one serving each day of fruits that are high in vitamin C—citrus fruits, melons, and strawberries are all good choices. Choose whole fruit over fruit juices, which don't contain as much healthy fiber.

Whole Grains

This group includes bread, pasta, hot or cold cereal, corn, millet, barley, bulgur, buckwheat groats, and tortillas. Build each of your meals around a hearty grain dish—grains are rich in fiber and other complex carbohydrates, as well as protein, B vitamins, and zinc.

Legumes

Legumes, which is another name for beans, peas, and lentils, are all good sources of fiber, protein, iron, calcium, zinc, and B vitamins. This group also includes chickpeas, baked and refried beans, soy milk, tofu, tempeh, texturized vegetable protein, peanuts, and peanut butter.

43. Reprinted with permission of Physicians Committee for Responsible Medicine.

Food Group	Number of Servings	Serving Size
WHOLE GRAINS	5 or more	½ cup hot cereal 1 ounce dry cereal 1 slice of bread
VEGETABLES	3 or more	1 cup raw ½ cup cooked
LEGUMES	2 to 3	½ cup cooked beans 4 ounces tofu or tempeh 8 ounces soy milk
FRUITS	3 or more	1 medium piece of fruit ½ cup cooked fruit ½ cup fruit juice

Round your diet out by including a good source of vitamin B_{12} (cobalamin). Most multivitamin pills include this nutrient, and many cereals are also supplemented with B_{12}.

Note: Use these serving numbers to help you plan healthy meals, not to get caught in a diet-like trap. These are guidelines. Rest assured, natural foods are nutritious foods. If you eat a variety of them, you will not ordinarily have to weigh, measure, or count servings. —V. M.

Reprinted with permission of Physicians Committee for Responsible Medicine

----

❧ AND IT TASTES GOOD, TOO! ❧

If you think whole grains, vegetables, legumes, and fruit sound too basic for fine dining, read the following buffet brunch menu from the news conference at which Physicians Committee for Responsible Medicine introduced the New Four Food Groups. I'm not recommending seven-dessert spreads and it's usually safest for food addicts to keep things simple. Nevertheless, lowfat, total-vegetarian food can dress up quite elegantly.

Buffet Brunch Menu

Creamy Banana Date Shake

·

*Chilled Melon Soup with
Berries and Roasted Pine Nuts*

·

*Assorted Vegetable Lasagna
Tortellini in Pesto Sauce*

·

*Ratatouille Ravioli with Shallot Confit
Red Bell Pepper Sauce*

·

Stuffed Grape Leaves with Rice and Almonds

·

Vegetarian Chili

·

*Potato, Leek, and Tofu Tart
Viennese Table
Orange Crème Brûlée
Lemon Trifle, Lemon Zest, and Strawberries
Piña Colada Mousse with Pineapple
Fruit Kebabs with Toasted Coconut
Apricot and Mango Sauce
Carrot Cake with Maple Syrup
Strawberry Shortcake*

◀ NUTSHELL NUTRITION: THE MACRONUTRIENTS ▶

If you're a food addict, you have probably read quite a bit about nutrition. (Even at ten I memorized nutrient charts while my friends read comic books.) You may, in fact, be quite fed up with the entire subject. If so, this mini-section is for you: nutrition in a nutshell or, to keep things lowfat, nutrition in a pea pod. We'll start with the big guys or macronutrients, carbohydrates, protein, and fats.

Carbohydrates

Unrefined carbohydrate foods are our foremost energy source and also the storehouses of other vital nutrients. Carbohydrate comes as either sugar or starch. Sugars are simple and can be utilized by the body almost immediately. Starches are broken down into sugars during the digestive process. Natural sugars are deliciously packed in fruit, with the highest concentration found in dried fruit. Starch is found in grains, vegetables, and legumes.

Refinement is good for social climbing but bad for carbohydrate nutrition. White sugar is the ultimate in this kind of refinement, so cut down on soft drinks and conventional baked goods. Use sweeteners like dates, fruit concentrates, maple syrup, and barley malt when you cook, but remember that all sweetness comes from sugar and even sweeteners from Mother Nature's kitchen can be overdone. Also, read labels. Corn syrup, brown sugar, raw sugar, fructose, dextrose, sucrose, and lactose are all forms of sugar, so beware of any packaged food product with a concentration of one or more of these. (Ingredients are listed on the label in order of the amount contained in the product. Some manufacturers are clever, though, and may use two or three types of sugar so no single one has to be listed as the first or second ingredient.)

Highly processed grains—white flour, white rice, degerminated corn meal—have also been robbed of nutrients. In "enriched" foods, some nutrients are replaced, but enrichment is like having the person who steals your car give you bus fare. Stick with the whole grains and simple cereals, but beware of granola—it's usually high in fat and terribly sweet. Also note that even refined carbohydrates are generally superior to any fatty foods. You'd do better with vegetable chop suey over white rice than with sweet and sour pork, or with white flour pasta and marinara sauce than veal parmigiana.

Protein

The golden age of protein has passed—the days when we believed that eating lots of it would dissolve body fat and having it in shampoo could glue split ends together. People are accepting that protein is simply a nutrient necessary for, among other things, growth, tissue repair, and combatting infection. The RDA (Recommended Daily Allowance) in the United States for protein is sixty-three grams for an adult male, and fifty for a nonpregnant female. However, those figures are well above the recommendation from the World Health Organization of thirty-nine grams per day for a male, twenty-nine for a female. In fact, meeting either standard on a varied, natural, vegetarian diet is not difficult. It may actually be a good idea to avoid going over the RDA very often because calcium depletion and kidney damage are among the problems that have been linked with excess protein consumption.

Amino acids are the units that make up protein. Eight of them, called the essential amino acids, must be supplied by the diet. It was formerly believed that only animal foods provided complete protein, i.e., all the essential amino acids, and that the only way vegetable foods could be made sufficient was to combine foods (generally grains and legumes) at the same meal to create an amino acid profile that looked like that of meat. This is not necessary. Simply eat a variety of foods throughout the day and in the diet overall. Although there are many vegetarian foods that are concentrated proteins—peanuts, dried beans and peas, soy products like tofu—these do not need to be emphasized. In fact, a cup of beans a day is plenty. And with a variety of whole, natural foods, you'll get ample protein even on a day you leave beans off the menu.

Fats

Fats provide warmth and a concentrated energy source, as well as the essential linoleic and linolenic fatty acids. Getting enough fat is not a problem in our society: the Standard American Diet averages forty percent of calories as fat, markedly above the recommended ten to twenty-five percent.[44] Saturated fats are found primarily in animal foods and butter, cheese, and meat, and in a few plant products, primarily coconut, chocolate, and palm oil. Unsaturated fats are abundant in vegetable oils, margarine, nuts, seeds, and avocado. Although saturated fats have been linked with high cholesterol levels and increased risk of heart disease, all fats are suspect factors in certain cancers. The safest course to take based on current knowledge is to keep total fat intake low. The most efficient way to do this is to eliminate fried foods and animal products and to be quite moderate in the use of higher fat plant foods such as peanut butter and oil-based salad dressings.

And Fiber, Too!

Fiber (or roughage) isn't really a nutrient, but this indigestible part of plants is important in digestion and elimination. A natural foods diet comprised of vegetables and salads, fruits, whole grains, and legumes is by definition a high-fiber diet, even without supplementary fibers such as wheat bran for bowel regularity or oat bran to lower cholesterol. (Besides, this is a zero-cholesterol diet which should eliminate the need for an extraneous cholesterol-lowering agent for most people.) Meat and most other animal products are virtually fiber-free. Fiber is also lost in processing, so try to choose whole fruits instead of fruit juice, whole grain bread instead of white, potatoes with their skins on, and so forth.

---

44. The conservative recommendations are usually to keep the diet under thirty percent fat, but overwhelming current evidence suggests that it should be well under that to ensure prevention of diet-related diseases for many people. Measuring the fat percentage in our diet on a daily basis, however, is impractical. The best way to keep fat intake at a safe level is to eat vegetables, fruits, whole grains, and legumes.

❦ NUTSHELL NUTRITION: THE MICRONUTRIENTS ❧

When it comes to vitamins and minerals, small is mighty. They don't take up much space in your body, but they are important. The Love-powered diet is like a health food store: it's full of vitamins and minerals. And when you consider that nutrition is still a relatively young science with more vital food components probably yet to be isolated, it is especially important to choose natural foods that haven't sacrificed their best parts to the miller or the cannery.

Minerals

Are body-building elements which also aid in digestion and temperature regulation. Among the major ones are:

Iron. *Needed by the blood for its oxygen supply, this mineral also aids in disease-resistance and red blood cell formation. Iron is found in leafy greens (collards, kale, broccoli), legumes (chickpeas, broad beans, limas), and other foods including whole grains and fruits, dried fruits in particular. Consuming a vitamin C-rich food along with an iron-rich food increases iron absorption by the body. The Recommended Dietary Allowance for iron is 10 milligrams a day for men, 15 milligrams a day for women.*

Iodine. *A tiny but essential amount (100 to 300 micrograms) is needed for energy production and proper functioning of the thyroid gland. It's added to iodized salt but is also abundant in sea vegetables (kelp, dulse, nori) and in vegetables grown in coastal areas with significant levels of iodine in the soil.*

Calcium. *Bone and tooth formation, blood clotting, muscle contraction, and nerve transmission require calcium. Because high protein intakes deplete the body's calcium stores, people with an adequate but modest protein intake (such as a natural foods, vegetarian diet provides) are believed to require less calcium than meat-eaters do. 1,200 milligrams a day of calcium is the current American RDA for young people eleven to twenty-four; 800 milligrams is recommended for people ages twenty-five to fifty. The World Health Organization's recommendation, however, is only 500 milligrams per day. Foods rich* in calcium include green leafy vegetables (collards and kale top the list), sea vegetables, nuts such as almonds and filberts, legumes such as chickpeas and pinto beans, and tofu cultured with calcium sulfate.

Phosphorus. *Phosphorus is used in a variety of body processes including energy production, but phosphorus is mainly calcium's right-hand mineral, important in bone and tooth development. Phosphorus is widely available in foods, and meeting the 800-milligram RDA for adults is not a problem. Rich sources include whole grains, legumes, peanuts, and peanut butter.*

Magnesium. *Required for the body's acid–alkaline balance and for blood sugar metabolism, magnesium is part of the nutrient package of peanuts, almonds, legumes such as soy and lima beans, millet, wheat, and rye. The RDA range for adults is 300–350 milligrams.*

Potassium. *Potassium is necessary for proper functioning of the heart and other muscles, and for nerves. You can find it in sea vegetables, soy and lima beans, dried apricots, sunflower seeds, and prunes.*

Sodium. *Sodium is lost in sweat, urine, and feces and is replaced by foods eaten, but most people get far too much. Table salt is the recognized source of sodium, but milk and its products, meats, canned vegetables, baked goods, and snack foods up the average intake considerably. Adequate sodium is provided by fresh vegetables. Use salt and soy sauce with a light hand.*

Selenium. *A trace mineral with antioxidant properties, selenium is a component of whole grains, broccoli, nutritional yeast, and the humble onion.*

Zinc. *Needed for proper growth, reproduction, and wound healing, zinc is in oatmeal, peanuts, peas, dried beans, and even popcorn. One study showed phytates in whole grains to inhibit zinc absorption, but this has not been evidenced clinically.*

Vitamins

Present in only small amounts but are vital to normal metabolism. They are either fat-soluble (vitamins A, D, and E) or water-soluble (vitamins B and C), the latter are more easily lost through careless preparation. Prolonged soaking and boiling are vitamin murderers; steam, bake, and stir-fry when you can. Turn leftover cooking water into soup stock. Better yet, eat raw foods whenever possible. A good salad—leaf or romaine lettuce instead of pale iceberg—is a vitamin pill with dressing.

Vitamin A. For healthy skin, eyes, and respiratory tract, think yellow and dark green: sweet potatoes, carrots, cantaloupe, dried apricots, kale, collards, spinach. The RDA is 800 micrograms for adult males, 1,000 micrograms for females.

Vitamin B complex. Needed for digestion, protein breakdown, and nervous system functioning, the "Bs" aren't called complex for nothing. They're a conglomerate of vitamins. Nutritional yeast (a fortified and tastier form of brewer's yeast) is the classic vitamin B health food, but members of the B family also congregate in whole grains, wheat germ, and peanuts. Here's a B by B breakdown, including some of the richest sources of each:

B_1 (thiamine) contributes to a good appetite, blood building, and carbohydrate metabolism. Rich sources are brown rice, sunflower seeds, soybeans, and other legumes.

B_2 (riboflavin) contributes to antibody and red blood cell formation, cell respiration, and metabolism of all food elements. Good sources are almonds, whole wheat bread, wild rice, leafy greens, and legumes.

B_4 (niacin) is needed for cell metabolism and respiration as well as carbohydrate absorption. The niacin deficiency disease, pellagra, was common prior to the enrichment of refined grains. Good sources are brown rice, wild rice, peanuts, millet, collards.

B_6 (pyridoxine) contributes to antibody formation and hydrochloric acid production. Good sources are peppers, leafy greens, cauliflower, citrus fruits, potatoes.

B_{12} (cobalamin) is required by the nervous system and by the blood (in miniscule but essential amounts). Since it is produced by microorganisms, most people can probably get all they need from the microbes that live in the mouth and intestines. Because B_{12} does not reliably occur in vegetable foods, the wise course for a total vegetarian is to take a supplementary B$_{12}$ tablet to meet the RDA of 2 micrograms or to regularly use foods fortified with cobalamin.

Vitamin C. *Involved in collagen production, digestion, healing, and resistance to infection, vitamin C gets to the table in citrus fruits, cantaloupe, strawberries, bell peppers, cabbage family vegetables, and Irish potatoes. The RDA for adults is sixty milligrams per day, although a substantial body of research indicates that a higher intake is optimal.*

Vitamin D. *The sunshine vitamin is essential for teeth and bones so it is especially critical for children and pregnant women; it's also needed for calcium metabolism and heart action. Although dairy products and margarine are fortified with it, nature meant for us to get vitamin D from the action of sunlight on the skin. Since most of us don't get sun all year, vitamin D is stored in our tissues.*

Vitamin E. *Vitamin E is an antioxidant that regulates destructive oxidizing of cell membranes and vitamin A. It's widely available, particularly in whole grains, wheat germ, sweet potatoes, leafy greens, and navy beans. The RDA is eight milligrams daily for adult females, ten for males.*

—✠—

EIGHT

Eating to Live

In this chapter, we'll be pragmatic, dealing with grocery carts and restaurant menus, and with the culinary basics of natural, vegetarian
dining. This should not lead you to believe that we have left the spiritual part of the Love-powered diet for something else. With a well-
tuned inner life, you can see miracles in the mundane, the Creator in
the created, the profound in the practical.

Having started on an inner path means that you're loving yourself,
others, and life more and more. One way to express that love is with

the food choices you make—the quality of fuel you offer your body, the manufacturing and agricultural practices you support. You've seen how a Love-powered diet can make an important contribution to your physical well-being, the role it plays in keeping weight at a comfortable level, and how a ripple effect from it can go beyond your personal health and happiness to help create a gentler society and a healthier planet.

The spiritual exercises and attitude revisions we dealt with earlier can make it possible for you to live serenely without abusing food. Conversely, the way you eat can affect your mental and spiritual life. When you're eating the purest, most healthful foods available to you, you feel good about your body, your thinking is more lucid and your outlook more positive. Your interior life and your outward actions then complement each other. They meet full circle, so it's hard to say which was first.

Eating (destructively) has been the problem, but eating (constructively) is an essential part of solving it. For this reason, we need to talk about food. If you are a food addict, be sure you're in a good place internally for reading and thinking about food right now. As long as you are in the state of spiritual fitness that *Alcoholics Anonymous* refers to as "a position of neutrality, safe and protected,"[1] you can open yourself without fear to all the useful information you'll need. In that frame of mind, you aren't fraternizing with the enemy in learning about a better way of eating and trying out different foods and cooking techniques. You are instead developing a new and healthier relationship with food.

Remember as we get into the specifics about particular Love-powered foods, about shopping, cooking, meal-planning, eating out, and the like, that we're going to be viewing food from a perspective that may be unlike any you've taken before. *We will not look at food only in terms of how it tastes, how much fat is in it, or how many vitamins and minerals it provides, but how we feel about it and how it makes us feel.*

Take, as an example, string beans. If you're going to use the fresh ones, they need to have their ends removed. It's tedious, but I'm convinced that such chores are far more meaningful than they appear,

---

1. *Alcoholics Anonymous*, p. 85.

because they speak of our connection with nature, a connection that is stabilizing and healing.

Of course it's easier to open a bag of frozen beans. They don't have any more calories than fresh ones, and nutritionally they're virtually identical. Sometimes saving minutes is a legitimate priority, but the price paid for the convenience is that we give up the tactile and participatory experience of taking the fresh option. We tend to think that aerobic exercise is the only activity that helps keep a body fit and trim. That's not so. Snapping beans and shelling peas do it, too, just in a different way. *They put us in a sort of psychic kinship with the foods we eat, with the soil, the seasons, the source of physical life and nourishment.* Binge eating is in direct opposition to this kinship, because it shuts us off from all these things.

◀ A GENTLE TRANSITION ▶

You will soon experience a lot of changes—changes in your outlook toward food as well as in your diet. Before we look at the dietary shift, let's work a little with change itself. Please get a piece of paper and a pencil or pen. We're going to make some lists.

First, jot down three really important, positive changes that you've made in your life, actions that in retrospect you're very glad you took. Now, think back to when each was just beginning. How was it? Did you love whatever it was without reservation, or was there a period of adjustment? Was your positive change (going off to college, moving to the country, making a mid-life career move, etc.) comfortable from the start, or did you have to get used to it?

My list of important, positive things is (1) living in London after I graduated from high school; (2) becoming a parent; and (3) giving up my regular magazine job to free-lance full-time. These are among the red-letter events of my life, turning points for which I'm deeply grateful. Nevertheless, when I arrived alone in the huge capital of a foreign country at the age of eighteen, I wanted to turn around and run back through customs in the other direction. When my daughter was born, I realized that not one of the fifty-seven books I'd read when I was pregnant had prepared me for the reality of caring for a tiny human being. And once I left the security of a steady job for the sink-or-swim uncertainty of self-employment, I felt that I'd joined a trapeze act that didn't use a net.

These separate and qualitatively different events took place over a twenty-year time span, yet each required patience and persistence from me for its richness and beauty to become apparent. You probably noticed this during the important, positive events in your own life. Now you're about to chalk up another important, positive thing as you adopt Love-powered eating. The change for you could be relatively minor—maybe you're already a vegetarian, but you haven't been able to let go of cheese and ice cream—or it may call for a ninety-degree turnaround in your eating habits. Whether subtle or startling in its particulars, however, this change will be significant. *Allow yourself a gentle transition.*

If choosing to eat in a way that expresses love to yourself and others is a commitment that grows from your deepest self, you'll realize that you're in this for the duration. You don't have to know everything right away. You don't have to be an expert. You only need to choose the very best foods you know of for today's three meals. Tomorrow, you'll know a little more and your choices then will reflect that.

I'd like to help you ease into this transition by reminding you of the Love-powered eating that you're already familiar with, that you already do. **There are times in your life, probably many such times, when you are not eating for a fix, when you eat some fresh, natural food and really enjoy it. That's Love-powered eating. You already know how to do it. We'll go from there and we'll build on that.** We can start by exploring the Love-powered food groups—fruits, vegetables, whole grains, and legumes—and some of the foods in those groups with which you're already acquainted.

Fruit—Nature's Candy Store

We'll begin with fruit because you eat fruit now and you probably like it. Nearly everybody does. It is possible to become so jaded by over-indulgence in refined sweets (candy, pastries, and the like) that the delicate flavors of fruit are no longer appealing. After a few days away from sugary foods, though, fruit becomes a real treat. It's sweet and delicious, a veritable vitamin factory, and virtually fat-free. Fruit makes an ideal breakfast, handy snack, or light dessert[2] that's always ready. You don't have to do anything to it, just enjoy.

Let's get back to that piece of paper. Write down your ten favorite fruits. That sounds like quite a few, but it won't be hard once you get started. Think of the exotic fruits you had on your trip to Hawaii. Remember that interesting melon you found at the greengrocer's last summer, and the wild strawberries you picked at your grandmother's so long ago. You'll find you already know some of nature's tastiest tidbits—and there are lots more where those came from. Now allow me to introduce you to my ten favorites:

Banana.[3] Most people aren't aware that there are more than a dozen varieties of banana, each distinct. In northern climates, our selection isn't terrific (a banana is a banana), but even these make my list because, when frozen, they turn a simple blender drink into something frothy and luscious. They can even become a treat that is astonishingly like ice cream! Use really ripe bananas (the skins need to be well-flecked with brown), peel them, and freeze in air-tight containers. If you have a clever appliance called the Champion Juicer (see "Good Food Gadgets" in the "Culinary Basics" section of this chapter), you can run uncut frozen bananas through with the "homogenize blank" in place for delectable soft-serve. As an alternative, chop the bananas in one-inch rounds before freezing and puree them in your food processor, using the metal blade. You will need to scrape down the sides with a spatula every so often until the banana is processed to soft-serve consistency.

Cherries. Cherries remind me of my dad, of visiting home and going with him to a certain produce merchant at the city market for the darkest, sweetest bing cherries in season. Because of their pits,

2. Some people notice digestive discomfort when they eat fruit with other foods. For them, it's best to have fruit *a cappella*. For more on the theory behind this, see *Fit for Life*, listed in Appendix A.

3. George Eisman, M.S., R.D., has pointed out an ethical problem in eating tropical fruits imported from Third World countries in his book *The Most Noble Diet*. Fruits grown for export often use land that could grow staple foods for the native population. The North American Vegetarian Society (Appendix C) stocks Eisman's book. A source for domestically grown tropical fruit that can be shipped direct to you is Starr Organic Produce, P.O. Box 561502, Miami, FL 33256.

cherries can't be bolted down. It seems to me like nature's way of saying, "I put a lot into these. Slow down and relish them."

Cantaloupe. Cantaloupe probably wouldn't make my top ten if it weren't for the smooth and tasty shakes that can be made from juicy, ripe ones. Chop a cantaloupe in cubes one- to two-inch square and put these in a blender with the smallest amount of water necessary to get the blender to liquify the fruit. It's really amazing how thick and creamy this turns out—an exquisite light breakfast or summer afternoon cooler.

Dates. Dates are rich relatives, very sweet and concentrated, and lack the high water content of most fresh fruits. They're too rich to eat as snacks (except for active children, athletes, and people trying to gain weight), but four or five big Medjool dates with lettuce leaves, celery, and a couple of crunchy Rome apples make my favorite light autumn lunch.

Mango. These are best when very ripe. You can often get them on sale when they look past their prime but are really just right for eating. Make a crosscut into the fruit starting on top and going one quarter of the way down the sides. You can peel a mango by hand from there. Have plenty of napkins nearby. Mangoes are juicy, messy, and delectable. (And like a banana, a peeled, ripe, frozen mango can be put through a Champion for a heavenly treat.)

Raspberries. I like how the British say "rahz-bries," and I like how these fragile, fragrant berries taste in any accent. I remember getting the summer season's last half-pint from a roadside stand in Indiana one summer and savoring every berry. That's when I realized that this slow savoring was the exact opposite of binge-eating. I have Indiana raspberries to thank for the insight.

Papaya. Papaya is an acquired taste, and it's true that most of those shipped to the north can't compare with the tree-ripened tropical gems. Still, if you let one completely ripen until it is yellow and spotted and has the same give as a ready avocado, it can be a real delight. (Don't eat even one of the black seeds that you'll scoop from the center. They're bitter.)

Persimmon. Life is too short to consider persimmons too expensive. I'd never tasted the world's most popular fruit until I was thirty and visited a resort in south Texas where custard-like persimmons were lunchtime specialties. I still get them often in late fall and winter, and although they do cost more than less dramatic fruits, I think the persimmons and I are both worth it. (Eat them when thy are *very* soft. When you think they're ripe, give them another couple of days.)

Strawberry fruit. This gets its name because the flowers on the tree look like strawberry blossoms. This tropical treat doesn't ship well so you probably won't have ready access to it and neither do I, but when we both get a dream vacation to somewhere that's always warm and sunny, we can look for these grape-sized white fruits that taste like caramels. Stuffed in half a papaya, they make a breakfast to write home about.

Watermelon. Watermelon is an air conditioner you eat. I never liked it much until I learned the secret of watermelon connoisseurship: eat it by itself, not with other foods. Its exquisite juiciness can't be appreciated in the company of other foods. (And people who have trouble digesting melon often find that eating it alone remedies that problem.) Be sure to eat *enough.* Its size is deceptive because a watermelon is mostly liquid. A terrific watermelon will be heavy for its size—that's the sweet juice weighing in!

Well, that was my ten. And there are also apples, oranges, grapefruit, tangerines, starfruit, honeydew, pomegranates, pineapple, kumquats, pears (prickly and otherwise), peaches, nectarines, apricots, grapes, kiwi, figs, plums, blueberries, blackberries, and more—fruits for every climate and all times of year.[4] You can see already that nature is *not* miserly. And we've only discussed *one* classification of the tasty offerings from her pantry. To finish up on fruit, here are some tips to remember.

---

4. For more on selection, storage, and preparation of fruit, see "All About Fruit" (pp. 75–79) in *The American Vegetarian Cookbook from the Fit for Life Kitchen* (see Appendix B). To learn more about unusual fruits and vegetables, I recommend *Uncommon Fruits and Vegetables, a Commonsense Guide,* by Elizabeth Schneider (New York: Perennial Library, Harper & Row, 1989).

Fruit Facts

- Fruit can be a de-*light*-ful breakfast, the perfect snack, or a dessert. (If eating fruit on top of other food doesn't agree with you, save your dessert for a couple of hours after the meal.)

- Eat fruit when it's fully ripe. Much fruit is picked green for shipping and, with the exception of citrus and apples, often needs to ripen after you get it home. Bananas ripen best in a brown paper bag, and placing a banana in such a bag with unripe papaya, avocado, or pears hastens their ripening as well. A lucite fruit ripening bowl also does the job while making a pretty centerpiece.

- Wash dirt, surface chemicals, and waxes from fruit (and vegetables) with a diluted detergent mixture (rinse well), or use a special cleaning product that's available for this purpose at natural food stores. (If produce is heavily waxed, you're better off peeling it.)

- Eat fruits whole most of the time instead of drinking juice. Juice is really a rich relative because its fiber has been removed and the natural sugars in juice can enter your bloodstream very quickly. When you do drink juice, dilute it by half with water (sparkling water and fruit juice over ice make a refreshing soda). Sip juice slowly, and prepare it fresh whenever possible. Citrus juicers, manual and electric, are inexpensive and easy to find in department and culinary stores. For information on machines that juice apples, grapes, etc., as well as vegetables, see the "Good Food Gadgets" on page 206.

- Other than for the occasional special dish (such as the poached apples and apple custard in the recipe section, Appendix B), eat fruit that is fresh and uncooked. Frozen, unsweetened berries and mixed fruit may be used in smoothies or when fresh fruit is not available, but use canned fruit—even juice-packed—only as a last resort. All canned foods have been heated.

- Because they are very sweet, treat dates and dried fruits as rich relatives. Particularly if you wish to release weight, have these only in moderation (half a dozen or so dates, figs, or prunes, or a handful of raisins a couple of times a week). Dried fruit is best soaked—reconstituted with water to more clearly resemble its fresh state—or save these rich foods for use in other dishes: to sweeten hot cereal, add to breads or muffins, or deliciously garnish a salad. If these sweets are binge foods for you, stick with fresh fruits.

· Plant a fruit tree. Plant two. Plant ten. There is a wonderful health retreat in Marathon in the Florida Keys called Club Hygiene[5] that had no more land than most suburban yards when its proprietor Douglas Graham, D.C., turned the property into a lush orchard with over 150 fruit-bearing trees in less than five years. Admittedly, we don't all live in the Florida Keys, but some kind of fruit tree will grow almost anywhere. Start with a dwarf tree that will mature rapidly so you'll have something to pick without too long a wait. Something momentous happens when you can get fruit from a tree you've planted. You deserve that experience and the earth needs every oxygen-producing tree she can get.[6]

◄ EVERYTHING'S COMING UP VEGIES! ►

When we discussed nutrition in Chapter 7, vegetables were mentioned time and time again. The leafy greens in particular are nutritional powerhouses. Many adults are still stuck in the six-year-old's notion that vegetables are "yucky." They also carry the stigma in many people's minds of being "rabbit food"—dietetic stand-ins for something you would really like. "I can eat ten carrots when I'm on a diet," I was told, "but when I'm not on a diet, I won't touch a carrot."

Let's face it. It takes some sophistication to truly appreciate vegetables. Children don't have it. The unimaginative who think of vegetables as canned peas and the lettuce on a burger don't have it either. But you do and we're going to explore that now. Think of a vegetable you honestly like. It needs to be one that you enjoy without cream sauce or gobs of butter, one that you don't eat fried, just raw or

5. The name comes from Natural Hygiene, a system of maintaining health through natural methods. Information on the American Natural Hygiene Society is given in Appendix C, "Some Helpful Organizations."

6. "Trees can, over time, remove large quantities of carbon dioxide (the main 'greenhouse gas') from the atmosphere. This makes planting a tree an effective way to fight the greenhouse effect. And it's easier than you might think." From *50 Simple Things You Can Do to Save the Earth*, p. 78. See pp. 78–79 of that book (listed in Appendix A) for more information.

steamed until it's bright and crisp. Write it on your paper as your favorite vegetable.

My favorite vegetable is broccoli. When I used to fast,[7] I didn't crave
the chips and candy bars that had got me in trouble, but I dreamed of
broccoli—lightly steamed with a squeeze of fresh lemon. Even then,
my subconscious knew the good stuff. Nowadays, I fix broccoli at
least once a week and order broccoli with garlic sauce every time I go
to a Chinese restaurant. My body seems to purr when it's had
broccoli.

How often do you eat your favorite vegetable? Is it one that can be
eaten both cooked and raw? Have you tried it both ways? Let's start a
new list. Write down ten other vegetables you like. Make two columns, one of five vegetables you like raw, or sun-cooked as I like to
think of it, and five you like cooked. (Some could be listed both ways,
but be sure to put down ten *different* vegetables altogether.) Here are
mine.

Favorite Home-Cooked Vegetables

1. *Asparagus.* Asparagus is a marvelous luxury. Try it slightly
steamed with a touch of herbal seasoning like Vegit or Mrs. Dash. It
reminds me of pay day.

2. *Fresh peas.* Eat them right from the pod, quickly steamed.

3. *Chinese wood ear mushrooms.* Chewy and hearty, wood ears
have a consistency that helps some people get over a yearning for
meat. I like them scored with crosscuts on top and sautéed in a little
oil and sherry with a dash of lemon juice and a few snips of parsley.
They can also be boiled for a minute and used in other vegetable or
grain dishes, soups, or stir-fries.

4. *Spaghetti squash.* These big, oval, yellow squash are lots of fun
since their meat, when cooked, is in strings like spaghetti. Scoop the
seeds from a halved squash, cut into quarters, and steam, or prick the
skin and bake whole. Serve with an herbal seasoning (plenty of
garlic) or a fresh tomato sauce.

---

7. Supervised fasting can be valuable in dealing with certain medical conditions and
it has a venerable spiritual history. I misused it, however, for quick weight loss.

5. *Kale*. Not only packing calcium, iron, and vitamin A, kale can be *delicious!* Dark, leafy greens have the reputation of being strong and bitter (maybe that's why salad bars often have kale *around* bowls for garnish instead of *in* them for food). Greens are misunderstood and underrated, though. Chop or shred kale (I use kitchen shears for this), steam in a vegetable steamer (see the "Good Food Gadgets" section on page 206) five or six minutes, and season with a little lemon juice, salt if you like, and add freshly ground pepper. (The same technique works for other greens—bok choy, chard, collards, endive, escarole, spinach. Steaming times vary a bit. See "A Steamy Romance—With Vegetables!" on page 189.

Favorite Sun-Cooked Vegetables

1. *Arugula*. This is no wimpy vegetable, but a Mediterranean contribution to a super salad that makes its presence known. Its taste can vary, sometimes in summer becoming quite hot and spicy, but giving a gourmet touch to any season's salad. Clean it well and use sparingly until you become an arugula aficianado.

2. *Fresh corn, cut from the cob*. When it's harvest time for corn and you can get it straight from someone's garden or just picked at a farmers' market, young corn is sweet and juicy and perks up a salad quite nicely. (Baking corn on the cob is another good idea. The result is a much more flavorful vegetable than when it's boiled. It also roasts beautifully over a fire or in coals on a picnic or camping trip.)

3. *Sweet red pepper*. Red bell peppers usually cost a little more than their more prominent green brethren, but the taste makes up for it. They're also such a wonderful color. A salad of Christmas-green spinach, a few shreds of purple cabbage, and bright red rings of sweet pepper feeds the eye before you pick up a fork.

4. *Cauliflower*. This is my favorite of crudités. So unlike the overcooked, grayish mush that passed for cauliflower in the school cafeteria, raw cauliflower is tasty without being strident and has a dandy crunch.

5. *Carrots*. I go through a peeler at least once a year because our household carrot consumption rivals that of Peter Rabbit's. Usually, I eat a carrot whole, but I'm also apt to shred a couple in the food

processor and use carrot instead of lettuce or sprouts on a sandwich; or make carrot-raisin salad. (You don't need mayonnaise for this— just mix shredded carrots with raisins and toss with a little pineapple juice and, optionally, a handful of sunflower seeds.)

I'm a fan of carrot juice as well. Like fruit juices, it's sweet and lacks fiber, but it's packed with betacarotene and energizing enzymes. Carrot juice is also the tasty base for making blends with less sweet vegetable juices. Carrot/beet and carrot/celery/parsley are wonderful. When I drink them, I feel as if I'm doing something really special for myself. Vegetable juices are best right from the juicer and drunk slowly. A stemmed glass doesn't hurt either.

Sun-cooked (raw) vegetables must be fresh in order to be palatable. I'll admit to cooking sagging spinach, yellowing broccoli, and carrots on the limp side when they would never have done for a salad or as crudités. You've probably done the same thing. There's nothing wrong with "waste not, want not," but it goes to show that vegetables that are delicious raw are literally the cream of the crop.[8]

Now we each have lists of our ten favorite vegetables to include in salads, on relish trays, steamed as side dishes, or mixed in casseroles and stir-fries. Starchy vegetables like potatoes, yams, and winter squash have enough substance to be entrées on their own. Following a salad with a steamed vegetable platter served with rolls or rice is a lovely meal, particularly in late summer when garden vegetables are most abundant. A salad itself can be a main dish when a heavier food like pasta, brown rice, or garbanzos is included in it; and hot vegetable soup with your own cornbread or bran muffins makes a fine winter lunch or late supper.

If your thumb has the slightest hint of green, consider doing a little gardening. Use fresh vegetables as often as possible; get the freshest-looking ones you see. Stay away from canned vegetables. They are overcooked before they ever see your stove, and most are heavily salted. *Experiment* with vegetables! For every one you're not too fond

8. Uncooked foods have many benefits. A fascinating exploration of these is provided in *Raw Energy*, by Leslie and Susannah Kenton (New York: Warner Books, 1984). As an all raw "cookless" book, I suggest *Light Eating for Survival*, by Marcia Acciardo, P.O. Box 702 Fairfield, IA 52556 (21st Century Publications, 1978), ring-bound and including charming illustrations, many by Peter Max.

of, there will be two or more that become your perennial favorites. Choose vegetables for their color, texture, nuances of flavor, or even the way they feel—don't forget the joy of snapping beans! "Culinary Basics" on page 174 contains information on making soup stock from vegetables, baking and stuffing the perfect potato, steaming vegetables, growing sprouts, and "The Art of the Salad.")

◀ GRAINS WHOLE AND HEARTY ▶

Grains are the food that let you know you ate. Whole grains are especially satisfying. They're substantial. You have to chew them. And when you chew grains, the digestive process starts right there in your mouth. The starches break down into their component sugars and the whole wheat bread or brown rice you're eating tastes heavenly.

If you've nearly always eaten refined grains like white rice and white flour products, the natural grains may at first seem tough or coarsely textured. Don't feel that you have to change to eating all your grains as whole grains overnight. There will probably always be times at restaurants or in social situations when only refined grains are available. Unless the particular food is a binge provoker for you, it's okay. You're improving your diet, not engaging in an endurance trial.

Give yourself some credit. Maybe you already eat oatmeal every morning and you truly prefer whole wheat bread, but you can't stand the thought of brown spaghetti. You're already ahead of the game. Give yourself some time. It won't be long before most of the refined stuff will taste like puffed air. Once you think of grains as generally referring to the whole grains that give an appetite what it came for and send it on its way, it will be much easier for you to see grains as a main course.

Let's go back to the piece of paper. Write down three meals you like that have a grain entrée. You can include pasta, waffles or pancakes, a rice dish, fresh bread with soup, even a special sandwich. Write it down even if the way you eat it now is high in fat or has animal ingredients. For example, you're probably used to pancakes made with milk and eggs. You can, however, make great pancakes that contain neither and use whole wheat flour, too. Love-powered eating also makes pizza a grain-based entrée since a really good crust is essential for a top-notch dairyless pizza.

Recipes for many popular dishes are given in Appendix B. If you don't find a Love-powered version of your favorite food there, you're almost certain to come across one among the recommended cookbooks. Many of these will include whole grains which are used creatively in vegetarian cuisine for everything from salads to loaves and burgers to wholesome desserts.

There's probably a lot more variety in the grains available than you might think. In addition to the familiar ones like wheat, rice, oats, and corn, there are many unusual varieties, mostly found in stores that sell natural or gourmet foods. Experiment with an uncommon grain. Sometimes trying something new is a good exercise in risk-taking. Ruts have a way of making themselves deeper, and the same-old-food rut is one of the easiest to get out of. So make millet or kasha or quinoa for dinner. It will probably be a tremendous success. And what if it isn't? Peanut butter sandwiches were invented for just such exigencies.

Keep the following things in mind about the grains in Love-powered eating:

- You don't have to skimp on your portions. You won't be eating gluttonously, but you'll be able to have ample, restaurant-sized servings of pasta, enough rice to fill you up, and sandwiches that needn't be open-faced.

- The old proscription against eating two starches at a meal no longer applies. You may not want both rice and potatoes or oatmeal and toast, but you can have them.

- Promote grains from side dish to main course both in your thinking and in your meals. (Here we've been discussing grains, but remember that starchy vegetables like potatoes, yams, and winter squash, as well as the lowfat, high-carbohydrate chestnut, have entrée potential as well.)

- Start the switch from refined to whole grains by revisualizing them. When someone says "bread," for example, consciously replace white with whole wheat in your mental image.

- If you're afraid of grains (you think they're fattening, or you've often binged on bakery goods), be clear on the tremendous difference between solid, sustaining whole grains and empty carbohydrates—pale, lifeless breads, and the cakes and cookies that contain not only refined flour but refined sugar and plenty of fat as well. Unrefined grains are not apt to set off cravings, and they're only high in calories when accompanied by fats (as in fried rice, or a muffin made with eggs and butter).

When you eat out, having a refined carbohydrate dish (white pasta or white rice, for example) is a reasonable compromise, one you can expect to make from time to time. When you do, you are still very much in keeping with Love-powered guidelines. *This is one way that your eating can alter slightly to fit your life, instead of altering your life to fit your eating.*

For more details on selecting and working with whole grains, see "The Granary" section of "Culinary Basics" on page 200.

◀ THE LOVE-POWERED BEANSTALK ▶

Like whole grains, legumes are substantial foods. It's not difficult to think of lentil soup or baked beans or chili as a main course. Beans do carry the stigma of being poor folks' food, but they're delicious just the same. And what's wrong with a bargain? Unfortunately, beans also have to live down their reputation for causing intestinal gas. It's true that they can be a culprit in this way, but there are things you can try to mitigate this, such as presoaking beans and discarding the soaking water; eating beans in simple combinations (for example, in a meal with only salad and a non-starchy vegetable); spicing them with the herb savory believed to mitigate the problem; sticking with sprouted beans (see "Sprout Farming" on page 187); and using more easily digested soy products like tofu instead of whole beans.

In fact, with versatile soy products such as tofu, soy milk, and meaty tempeh you can make this major change for the better in your diet without bereaving the loss of many of the foods that you're used to. Soy products are higher in fat than other legumes, but their ability to masquerade as a variety of animal foods makes these somewhat rich relatives well worth knowing.

If there are some foods you really think you'll miss when you eliminate animal products from your diet, write them down. Chances are, there is a reasonable facsimile (probably a soy product) sold commercially, or one you can make yourself from recipes in the cookbooks listed in Appendix B. I can't read your "miss list" but I can let you know that there are hot dogs, hamburgers, cheeses, milk-like drinks, and even ice creams made from soy. The recommended cookbooks have recipes for everything from kebobs and chicken salad[9] to sauerbraten and Gefilte Tofu![10]

Do some research and see what you come up with. **The only foods you need to release are those that are harmful to you in some way: foods that you obsess over, that are nutritionally inferior, and that inhibit the clear head and clear heart you need to allow Love to enter your life. Beyond that, eat the foods you *like*.** You can probably get plenty of help in this regard from what is sometimes called in the Orient "honorable soybean, meat without bone." (See "Tofu 101" on page 198.)

Other legumes can find a place on your menus, too. You can learn about more varieties, and about cooking with legumes, in "Bean Cuisine" on page 195. For now, write on your sheet three bean dishes you like—even if you've never had them without meat. With plenty of herbs and spices, your pork and beans can be just as good without the pork. Split pea soup is a tasty winter warmer that doesn't need ham, and great chili is a matter of beans, sauce, and seasonings, not ground beef. Just write down your favorite bean dishes to remind yourself that you'd probably like to have them more often. (If you're curious about my list, it's Boston baked beans, taco salad with chili beans, and my mom's black beans and rice—all meatless and all really good.)

Remember the following facts about legumes:

- Dried beans and peas are solid and filling. They will help ease your transition from heavy foods and excess food to a lighter, Love-powered diet.

- Soybeans and most of the products made from them are higher in fat than other legumes. Use them to replace the even higher fat

---

9. "Kebobs!" and "'Stedda' Chinese Chicken Salad," p. 116 and pp. 118–19, respectively in *The American Vegetarian Cookbook from the Fit for Life Kitchen*, by Marilyn Diamond. See Appendix B.
10. "German Sauerbraten" and "Gefilte Tofu with Horseradish and Charoset Sauce," pp. 146–47 and pp. 49–50, respectively in *Friendly Foods, Gourmet Vegetarian Cuisine*, by Brother Ron Pickarski, O.F.M. See Appendix B.

animal foods you no longer eat, but don't eat them exclusively. You don't want to bypass the lower fat beans.

· Legumes are a concentrated protein source. For this reason, don't overdo them. A cup of legumes a day is about right.

· If you haven't cooked beans much before, you may want to look into prepackaged bean soups, and rice and bean combinations that come with their own seasoning packets.

· It's okay to use canned beans, but if you need to keep your sodium intake especially low, you will want to drain and rinse them.

· Most bean dishes at nonvegetarian restaurants have some kind of pork in them, and some Mexican restaurants still use lard in their refried beans. Ask before you order.

◀ PUTTING IT TOGETHER ▶

When your pantry is filled with vegetables, fruits, whole grains, and legumes, you'll be ready for delicious meals that will nourish your body and free your mind to pursue all the inedible—and, in fact, incredible!—joys of life. Meal planning will not be a major issue. Helen Nearing, a modern Thoreau in her philosophy of simple living, writes of her version of Love-powered eating:

> Our menus are simple, but vary within the daily pattern; some fruit or fruit juice and our own herb tea for breakfast; a hearty vegetable soup, with boiled grains, peanut butter, honey and apples for lunch; a big salad, some cooked vegetable from the garden and a fruit dessert for supper. Every day the soup can be different. The grain can be millet, buckwheat, oats, wheat or rye. The salad need never be the same. The vegetables vary with the season. Our dessert can be any of many fruits, raw or cooked. But the general pattern remains, so that the diet is uninvolved and the preparation uncomplicated.[11]

11. Helen Nearing, *Simple Food for the Good Life, a Collection of Random Cooking Practices and Pithy Quotations* (Walpole, NH: Stillpoint Publishing, 1980), pp. 20–21. Helen Nearing is one who has inspired me to investigate the less traveled road in my outlook toward life and in choosing an animal-free diet. A Renaissance woman who with her late husband Scott homesteaded in New England *twice*, Helen has celebrated nature and simple ways in *Wise Words on the Good Life* and other books. Her work has shown me that I can embrace nature and simplicity *in my own way*. I'm far from a back-to-the-land person and expect to remain so, but I can still appreciate my connection with the earth and with life's simple pleasures.

I, too, have a basic, nonrigid food plan providing me with some structure so I don't have to think much about food. I have fruit for breakfast—a smoothie more often than not. Other times, I make fresh orange juice when I get up and later on have a more substantial meal: hot cereal with dried fruit, cold cereal with soy milk, a bran muffin, or toast with fruit preserves. On Sundays or holidays, I make pancakes or French toast (egg-free, dairy-free recipes are in Appendix B).

When I'm really organized, I make a big salad right after breakfast so it's ready for lunch. I put in garbanzo beans or avocado and raisins so there's more to the salad than simply greens, and I eat it with a roll or crackers. Much of the time, I'm *not* that organized and don't think about lunch until I'm ready to eat it. Then I have leftovers from the previous night's dinner, or I make a sandwich (a mixture of raw and sautéed vegetables in a tortilla is quick and good), or I heat some soup. I usually make a big pot of soup on the weekend to have available throughout the week, or every now and then I'll have canned soup with whole grain rolls, raw vegetables, and bean or tofu dip. These foods travel well, too: soup in a thermos, salad in Tupperware®, sandwiches in waxed paper with tomato packed separately to avoid soggy bread.

Dinner is almost always a large salad, an entrée based on whole grains, legumes, or potatoes, and a steamed vegetable. Sometimes there's dessert—apple crisp or a nondairy "ice cream"—but not too often. You may be saying, "Rolls! Potatoes! Apple crisp! That's okay for you: you're not trying to lose weight. What about me?" Let me assure you that this is precisely how I did lose weight. It was never dieting, though, because with the generous assistance of unconditional Love my eating went from inappropriate to appropriate. I ate the food needed by a person with a normal-sized body and my body became normal-sized. I eat the same way today and it remains a normal size. Although you are likely to release weight quite easily after you begin to eat this way, it is not a quick weight-loss scheme. It is a *way of life* that is meant to be *for life*.

◄ OUT TO EAT ►

A frequent occurrence for most people these days is going out to eat. The Love-powered diet accommodates this. Ethnic restaurants are the most fun because the cuisines of Italy, China, Thailand, India, Ethiopia, and the Middle East feature numerous, totally vegetarian dishes. Moreover, you can eat well at almost *any* restaurant. Salad bars are easy if you just avoid anything laden with mayonnaise or overly oiled. Cafeterias are fine with their salads, vegetables, and breads; and potato bars are in many mall food courts and fast-food restaurants. Steak houses always have baked potatoes and some kind of salad, and most diners do, too. The fast-food Mexican places can do bean burritos without cheese, and at least one of the popular burger chains will make a vegetarian rendition of their big sandwich.

At elite restaurants, the chef and other personnel will usually go out of their way to provide you with a vegetable plate or special pasta dish or salad even if it's not on the menu. Wherever you're eating, graciously ask for what you need and expect to get it. You can reserve a pure vegetarian meal when you make airline reservations. (Reconfirm this twenty-four hours before the flight.) You can also make an advance request for a vegetarian meal for almost any banquet or catered dinner.

I've had very acceptable meals in some very diverse situations. Once I attended a posh dinner reception after a movie premier to write about the event for a magazine. I'd phoned the country club ahead to ask for vegetarian food. When the vegetable plate arrived (looking like the cover of a fine cookery magazine) my black-tied tablemates were obviously disappointed with their filet mignon. Several asked the waiter if there were any extra vegetable plates so they could make a trade!

In a completely different sociological environment, I was hungry in the midst of a journey by bus through Florida. My dinnertime layover was at a little depot and the only food available was provided by a hot dog vendor outside. He made me a hoagie sandwich of sorts: mustard, ketchup, relish, pickles, onion, and shredded lettuce piled on a frankfurter roll. It wasn't the Ritz, but it had a certain charm.

And some years ago on an extended car trip through the rural West, I was getting awfully tired of eating potatoes, toast, and less-than-fresh salads. I wandered into a truck stop in the wilds of Montana and right there on the menu in bold print it said, "Avocado and Sprout Sandwich on Dark Rye Bread." Given the setting, it was almost a surrealistic sandwich, albeit much appreciated.

Whether you're eating in Love-powered fashion or not, you will have some most enjoyable experiences in restaurants and some that aren't so great. A bonus of the Love-powered way is that whether dining out is superb or so-so won't matter very much. **You will find that as your attitude becomes more and more empowered by Love, food may be more delicious than ever, but it will definitely be less important.**

◄ AMONG FRIENDS ►

When you eat with other people, those people and the conversation you share will be the highlights of the occasion, regardless of what is served. Food prepared for guests needs to be simple and inviting. By and large, people enjoy this kind of food. Even those who have no desire to revamp their own style of eating appreciate a natural, vegetarian meal as a change of pace. (I think it also makes them feel that they've done something nice for their bodies, which indeed they have.)

When you're invited to be a guest for a meal in someone else's home, know that you've been invited because you're liked, not because you'll clean your plate! Let your friend know that your dietary needs are different now and make it clear that you don't need special treatment. Salads, breads, and grain and vegetable side dishes are usually more than ample at formal dinners; and if the affair is informal— a buffet or a pot luck—select what you want and leave what you don't. Bringing a dish to share is not always appropriate, but most of the time it's a welcome gesture.

People are quite understanding today about others' dietary preferences. Give your friends and relatives the opportunity to be understanding of yours. Although I can't verify it statistically, my experience and that of people I know has been that in changing to Love-powered eating, the social and logistical difficulties that were expected to crop up often actually happened quite seldom. *When you adopt a Love-powered diet because you love yourself and every living thing enough to do that, maintaining it is simply not difficult.* I think it has something to do with commitment, a stand that in itself carries astonishing power. During a period of uncertainty in my life, my friend Sue shared a quote with me that I've really cherished: "When one truly commits oneself, then Providence moves, too." It's never failed: my commitment has to come first, then doors open that I never knew were there.

Your commitment in this case is not to stick to this diet no matter what. Your commitment is to be motivated by Love—no matter what. You'll see the importance of this in your dealings with those closest to you. If you have a family or a close relationship with another person, you won't be alone when you alter the way you eat. Ideally, your spouse or parents or others with whom you live will read this book and come to realize why you're making the changes you are. Perhaps they will want to adopt Love-powered eating for themselves.

Or they may see this as one more diet, one more phase. They might be threatened by changes they see in you, even those that they've asked you to make, such as losing weight. Your new way of eating could seem extreme to them and they may let you know that they think you've gone too far. If so:

- Get the support you need elsewhere
- Eat the way that's best for you
- Remember to be grateful daily for the people you love, even when they aren't as supportive as you'd like
- Refrain from the urge to try to convert everybody

As we said before, in talking about the inner transformation you're undergoing, your life will speak for you. This is true of your new way of eating as well. Whether it's your trimmer body, your higher energy level, or your improved state of mind, Love-powered living and Love-powered eating will *show*. People will want what you've got.

In the meantime, accept the people around you and be willing to put up with some inconvenience. If another family member usually does the cooking, share your needs with that person and make it clear that you don't want to make extra work for him or her. Be willing to cook some of your own food. Offer to take over kitchen duties a couple of nights a week: the regular cook will get a break, and you'll get to introduce Love-powered eating to your family without pushing it.[12]

12. Children as well as adults can be well-nourished and grow properly on a starch-based, varied, natural foods diet. For more information, see *Pregnancy, Children & the Vegan Diet* by Michael Klaper, M.D. (available from the American Vegan Society, see Appendix C), and *The Vegan Diet During Pregnancy, Lactation, and Childhood* by Reed Mangels, Ph.D., R.D. (from The Vegetarian Resource Group, Appendix C).

If you wear the chef's hat most of the time and your family expects meat at dinner, serve it with love. For the last several years of her life, I cared for the elderly woman who had helped raise me. She did not eat much meat, but at times she got a hankering for bacon or sardines or stewed chicken. Although I was committed to Love-powered eating for myself, I fixed those things for her when she asked for them. When she was in the hospital at the age of eighty-seven, she told me she realized that being vegetarian was important to me, that preparing her meat had probably been hard, and that she had appreciated it. Shortly after that, she passed away.

Some people could say that I would have shown more love to her by giving her healthy vegetarian food without exception. Maybe they're right. In the same situation today, I might do just that. But at the time I was following my heart. What she told me just before she died had a lot more to do with that intangible aspect of the human heart than with bacon or sardines.

When you are healthy and happy and free from obsession, you'll also be freer to love your family and your friends and yourself. If you're not yet healthy and happy and obsession-free, love your family and your friends and yourself anyway; it will help you get there. Love the foods that nourish your body and the life that nourishment provides you. Love your fullness and your emptiness. Most of all, love God, by whatever name you choose, and see your emptiness filled and your fullness redeemed. When you love like this, you'll soon discover that you're no longer eating to fill a bottomless pit, to solve a hopeless problem, or squelch a nameless fear. You're eating to *live*.

❦ CULINARY BASICS ❧

Culinary Basics Table of Contents

To Market, To Market
Natural Foods Glossary
Going Organic
The Art of the Salad
Sprout Farming

A Steamy Romance—With Vegetables!

Soup Stock

The Perfect Potato (and Toppers)

Sandwich Ideas

Bean Cuisine

Tofu 101

The Granary

Fat Zappers

Good Food Gadgets

Kitchen Ecology

This booklet-within-a-book will provide you with the background to shop for, prepare, and serve the Love-powered foods that you will feel good about eating. These foods also have the potential to improve your overall health and to encourage your fix-free lifestyle. Take as much or as little information as you need to make eating naturally a natural part of your life. The basics are here.[13] For more, see the selected recipes and recommended cookbooks in Appendix B. If you have no interest in cooking, or if you want to keep things very simple, there will be some material here that won't apply to you. Pick and choose.

Your personal cooking style can be part of your solution just as it was part of your problem. *Food addicts who are good cooks let their disease take over that talent. They spend most of their time in the kitchen and specialize in preparing their binge foods. In recovery, however, people with a gift for food preparation can use it to put together beautiful, healthful, Love-powered meals for themselves and those they love. Since they're cooking because they want to and not because an obsession is forcing them to, the kitchen becomes one of many places for them to express creativity, artistry, and love.*

On the other hand, there are food addicts who detest cooking. They stock up for binges at convenience stores and fast-food eateries, and in a pinch can binge on anything in the kitchen that requires no prep-

---

13. Some of the information here on marketing, natural foods, cooking grains and beans was originally used in an article I wrote for *Vegetarian Times*, "Passing Go, a Beginner's Guide to Vegetarian Cooking," January 1990. This information is used with the permission of *Vegetarian Times*.

aration. When these people get well, they're not apt to become gourmet chefs. They can turn their lack of interest in cooking to an advantage, emphasizing simplicity in their meals. In her book Simple Food for the Good Life, Helen Nearing sums up the fancy versus fussless cooking debate from the viewpoint of one who prefers the fussless route:

> Make your meals simple, simpler, simplest—quick, quicker, quickest. And in the time and energy you will save, write a poem; make music; sew a fine seam; commune with nature; play tennis; visit a friend. Keep drudgery out of your life. If you love cooking, it is not work for you or drudgery. That's fine. Go to it and enjoy the joy of cooking. But if it is drudgery, stop it, or lessen it; you will be able to eat well and then go and do your own thing.[14]

◄ TO MARKET, TO MARKET ►

You can put Love in your diet and be well nourished shopping only at your local supermarket. Hit the produce department first; you'll do most of your shopping there. Then make brief stops at frozen foods and other strategic points within the store. There will be entire sections you'll bypass—the butcher's counter, the aisles of foodless snack foods and soda pop. Grocery shopping will get much quicker and easier. You'll probably notice that your food bill will decrease markedly as well.

Although it's not mandatory, you will find that your meals will be more interesting if you get to know the stock of a good natural food store. This is where you're most likely to find vegetarian specialty items—soy milk, egg replacer to be used in baking, mixes for meatless burgers and chili, and a wider variety of grains and beans than are available at conventional grocery stores. You can also expect to find organically grown grains, beans, and produce. (See "Going Organic" on page 182.)

Some of the prices at natural food stores will seem high, but you will get value for your money and in many cases support small, care-

14. Helen Nearing, Simple Food for the Good Life, a Collection of Random Cooking Practices and Pithy Quotations, p. 23.

ful companies whose profit margin is meager for the quality they offer. In some cases, you can actually save money at a natural food store. In particular, when you buy grains, flour, and nuts from bulk bins, you can choose the exact quantity you want and avoid paying for expensive packaging.

A real money-saver for the energetic is a food co-op. There are storefront co-ops and private buying clubs that you can join. By working for the co-op a few hours a month, you can buy your food at a hefty savings. (Being part of a co-op is also a way to meet other people who are interested in living more naturally and healthfully.)

For now, though, we'll stick with the supermarket. Get yourself an imaginary shopping cart and we'll make the weekly grocery run. Here's your list. Don't feel that you would have to buy all of this on a real shopping trip! This is a sample list including most of the items called for in common vegetarian recipes, and I've stuck with those foods that are most widely available throughout the country. If there are other vegetables, fruits, whole grains, and legumes that you like, add them to the list. And if there are items listed that you don't like— or that are binge foods for you—make a different selection. (An asterisk indicates a rich relative.)

◄ SAMPLE SHOPPING LIST ►

Produce

Lettuce—leaf, romaine (iceberg is all right, but less nutritious)

Spinach

Alfalfa sprouts

Tomatoes

Cabbage, red or green

Celery

Bell peppers

Broccoli

Carrots

Mushrooms

Onions (scallions, too, if you like)

Potatoes for baking (new potatoes, too, if you want them)

Yams

Apples

Oranges

Bananas

Other fruits in season

Frozen Foods

Unsweetened frozen fruit

Fruit juice concentrate*

Frozen lemon juice

Vegetables of your choice (plain, not with fancy sauces)

Canned Goods

Tomato sauce, paste

Tomatoes

Beans—pintos, garbanzos, chili beans in sauce, vegetarian baked beans (these may contain sugar)

Soups (optional—most canned soups are quite salty. Choose those vegetable, lentil, and minestrone soups without chicken or beef broth.)

Packaged Food

Whole wheat bread (read the label—"wheat flour," "flour," and "enriched flour" all mean white; look for 100% whole wheat)

Brown rice (get regular and quick-cooking) and rice pilaf

Whole wheat flour (if you bake yeast bread; using part unbleached white flour may be a good transitional step)

Whole wheat pastry flour (for quick breads, muffins, etc.)

Aluminum-free baking powder (Rumford's is one such brand)

Oatmeal (quick or old-fashioned)

Dry cereal (look for whole grains and a low sugar content; avoid granola)

Whole grain pasta (noodles, spaghetti)

Rice cakes, whole grain crackers, and corn to pop

All-fruit jam or conserves* (these contain no added sugar)

Dried beans and peas: lentils, split peas, navy beans, or your choice

Natural peanut butter*, English walnuts*, slivered almonds*

Raisins*, other dried fruit* if desired (get it without sulphur dioxide)

Extra virgin olive oil*

Apple cider vinegar, mustard, natural soy sauce (look for reduced sodium tamari)

Real maple syrup* or, optionally, honey*

Herbal teas, Postum, or Pero (grain coffee substitutes), bottled waters

Herbs and spices of your choice (Mrs. Dash is a good salt-free seasoning; the most popular spices used in vegetarian cooking are garlic, freshly ground pepper, onion powder, basil, oregano, cumin, chili powder, curry, parsley flakes, and paprika—sweet Hungarian paprika is best)

Refrigerated Foods

Tofu* (a refrigerated food but likely to be found in produce section)

Corn and/or whole wheat tortillas (sometimes frozen)

Yeast (if you bake. Note that baking yeast and nutritional or brewer's yeast are entirely different and not interchangeable.)

◀ NATURAL FOODS GLOSSARY ▶

The fruits and vegetables with which you're already familiar are true natural foods, and a healthful diet doesn't demand a boundless repertoire of different grains and legumes. Nevertheless, becoming acquainted with some of the more unusual foods can give your meals welcome variety. Some of these, tofu for example, can also be used to create dishes reminiscent of those you no longer eat and may miss. A Love-powered food-style does not require that you eat these things (many of them are, in fact, rich relatives), but they are available at natural food stores for you to try.

Agar-agar. A vegetarian gelatin made from seaweed. (Regular gelatin is a slaughterhouse byproduct.) Agar comes in sticks or flakes (the flakes yield the most consistent results). Use it like ordinary gelatin; one tablespoon of flakes will gel one cup of liquid.

Barley malt.[15]   A liquid sweetener made from sprouted barley, similar in flavor to molasses. (Rice syrup is another natural sweetener, quite delicate.)

Buckwheat. A hearty, quick-cooking grain with an earthy flavor. It can be cooked whole as a breakfast cereal or as a substitute for rice; as a flour, it's most popular in pancakes.

Carob. A chocolate-like treat from the pods of the locust tree. It comes in powder form for baking or making cocoa-like drinks and is also made into candies. (Many of the candies are high in oil, however, and some contain sugar or milk.)

Egg replacer. Powder to be substituted for eggs in baking. Use one teaspoon egg replacer whisked with two tablespoons water for each egg called for. (Ener-G and Jolly Joan are brand names.)

Granular sweeteners. Date sugar is ground, dehydrated dates. It has a full-flavored taste, something like dark, brown sugar. Fructose, generally derived from corn in spite of its name, looks and tastes like white sugar but is metabolized more slowly. Sucanat® is made from sugar cane juice that's been dehydrated and milled into a powder. It is richly flavored and very good in quick breads and bran muffins. (See footnote 15.)

Millet. Little, round, golden grains that cook up light and fluffy. Use as you would rice at dinnertime, as a hot breakfast cereal, or as a base for other dishes such as vegetarian loaves and burgers. (And throw millet instead of rice at newlyweds since it won't harm the birds who eat it.)

---

15. Remember that all sweeteners are sweet, natural or not. If you binge on sugary foods, proceed cautiously with any concentrated sweetener.

Miso. *Salty, fermented paste made from cooked, aged soybeans and sometimes from grains. Thick and spreadable, it's used for flavoring a wide variety of dishes and for making soup bases.*

Nutbutters. *Bread spreads from almonds, cashews, sunflower seeds, etc., as well as from peanuts. These are definitely rich relatives and very high in fat, but they can be used in moderation and in the preparation of other dishes. One you'll see called for in recipes fairly often is* tahini, *made from sesame seeds.*

Nutritional yeast. *Imparts a sharp, cheesy flavor to sauces, soups, casseroles. It can also be sprinkled on toast, popcorn, or spaghetti. Yeast flakes taste much better than powder. Either form is rich in B-complex vitamins, and many brands are fortified with vitamin B_{12}.*

Quinoa *(pronounced KEEN-wah). A round, sand-colored grain with a mild, nutty taste and a fascinating history going back to the ancient Incan culture. This cooks quickly.*

Ramen noodles. *Dry, wavy noodles that need only be boiled or steamed a few minutes to reconstitute their texture and be ready to eat. They come in packages with seasonings included for a nearly instant meal.*

Raw cashews. *Nuts, or, technically, the fruit of the cashew tree. Raw cashews are white and quite unlike roasted, salted cashews. High in fat, these are rich relatives like all nuts, but they're extremely versatile and relatively small amounts of them can be used to make "milk," "white sauce," and a variety of other dishes. Buy the pieces rather than whole cashews to save money.*

Seitan. *Chewy, high-protein food made from baked or boiled wheat gluten. Seitan tastes much like meat when used in stews, casseroles, or barbecued on a bun.*

Soy milk. *Milk-like beverage made from soybeans. The label will usually say "soy beverage" (not milk). This comes in liquid or powdered form. The fat content varies; look for the "lite" varieties.*

Tamari. *Natural soy sauce, fragrant and flavorful. Traditional ta-mari is wheat-free. Soy sauce made from soy and wheat is called "shoyu." These seasonings are very salty. Reduced-sodium tamari is less so.*

Tempeh. *A fermented soyfood with Indonesian heritage. Tempeh is very meaty in texture, barbecues beautifully, and is a natural for chili. (Like all soy products, it's fairly high in fat.)*

Tofu. *Soybean curd that's made its way from Chinese restaurant menus to most supermarkets. This white cake is virtually flavorless on its own so it takes on the character of the condiments used with it. It can serve as the "meat" in a stir-fry, the "sour cream" in stroganoff, the "cream cheese" in cheesecake. It's not a lowfat food, but it's much lower in fat than the cheese, mayonnaise, etc., it often fills in for. (See "Tofu 101" in this section for more ideas.)*

Wheat-free breads and pastas. *Breads, noodles, and spaghetti made from rice, rye, corn, and other grains. Wheat is a common al-lergen and many people are sensitive to wheat gluten. Natural food stores stock breads, crackers, and pastas that contain no wheat.*

◄ GOING ORGANIC ►

One way to show some extra love to yourself, other people, wildlife, and the earth is to purchase some organically grown foods. If you have some resistance to this idea, believe me: I held out on it for a long time. It seemed to me that only health fanatics, leftover hippies, and the people my grandmother used to say had "more money than sense" would pay the usually high price for organic groceries. I figured I was doing all right with regular food.

That was before I realized that synthetic insecticides, herbicides, and fertilizers weren't "regular" until some fifty years ago. Chemi-calized agriculture is a recent phenomenon that grew after World War II. (The pesticide parathion, for example, was developed by the Nazis as a lethal nerve gas. It's sixty times more toxic than DDT, but still applied around the world to grains, produce, and cotton.) And although the use of insecticides in agriculture has increased twelvefold over the past thirty years, damage to crops from pests has doubled during this time.

Research from France now suggests that some ammonia fertilizers and certain pesticides may prevent plants from absorbing micronutrients. "This not only makes them less nutritious," says agricultural economist Terry Gips, president of the International Alliance for Sustainable Agriculture,[16] "but it weakens the plant much like an immune deficiency, so insects can come to affect the weaker plants. It's a catch-22: the more you use, the more you have to use."

But consumers can opt for the organic alternative. Gips offers the following reasons for making the switch:

1. Personal health. *Conventionally grown food contains residues of various pesticides. A 1984 Natural Resources Defense Council study found forty-four percent of California's fresh produce contained residues of nineteen of these, including dieldrin and DDT, proven carcinogens.*

2. Social justice. *Nursing mothers in Central America have DDT in their breastmilk at levels forty-two times World Health Organization standards as a result of aerial spraying and residues in food. In the United States, the National Cancer Institute has found that farmers in Nebraska and Kansas who were exposed to the herbicide 2, 4-D run a six times greater risk of developing a rare form of cancer, nonHodgkins lymphoma.*

3. Wildlife protection. *Runoff from agricultural chemicals concentrates in ponds, contaminating the food and water of migrating waterfowl and resulting in deformities.*

4. Ecology. *Farming with sustainable, organic methods has many ecological advantages.*

Organic Methods save energy *(synthetic pesticides and fertilizers are made from petrochemicals—petroleum).*

Organic Methods do not contaminate ground or surface water. *Synthetic fertilizers cause nitrates, which break down*

---

16. A telephone interview with Gips (February, 1991) provided the factual information for this section. He is also the author of *Breaking the Pesticide Habit—Alternatives to Twelve Hazardous Pesticides* (Malaysia: International Organization of Consumers' Unions, 1990). Contact the International Alliance for Sustainable Agriculture at 1701 University Avenue S.E., Minneapolis, MN 55414.

into carcinogenic nitrosamines, to enter ground water. A 1990 U.S. Environmental Protection Agency study showed over fifty percent of wells tested to contain nitrates.

Organic Methods cause far less soil erosion. *Organic farmers rotate crops which produces richer soil. Their natural nitrogen fertilizers also make soil stronger, unlike artificial nitrogen which breaks down humus, making it susceptible to loss from wind and rain. "Five bushels of topsoil are lost for each bushel of corn conventionally grown," says Gips. "This is not sustainable."*

5. Economics. *Economics of scale in transportation and marketing means that the more people buy organic foods, the less those foods will cost. And every additional customer helps create the demand that will encourage more farmers to join the 50,000 in the United States who already farm organically.*

Natural food stores carry organically grown grains, nuts, legumes, and often fresh fruits and vegetables. Food co-ops make these available at a lower cost. Organic produce and some other foods are available at select supermarkets, as well. Demand creates supply. Ask for organic.

Look for foods labeled "certified organic." The word "natural" has no legal definition. It's usually applied to products with no synthetic colorings, flavorings, preservatives, or other artificial additives. That's good, but it says nothing about the way the food was grown. "Certified organic" means that an independent monitoring agency has inspected a farm and determined that no synthetic fertilizers or pesticides have been used there in the past three years, and that the farmer practices good soil management.

Now I can't tell you that you'll lose more weight or eat less obsessively when you fill your market basket organically. I do happen to believe that organically grown foods taste better. Maybe that's just because I like the way I feel about myself when I eat them. Or maybe some of the special care and attention that the farmers give the soil comes through in the rice and the carrots and the apples.

I also find that, for me at least, choosing organic foods seems to put me in closer touch with nature, with the land, with my part in all that is natural. Feeling connected in this way brings with it a balance that is antithetical to obsessing over anything. If paying an extra forty cents a pound for tomatoes can give me that, I'm getting quite a bargain.

THE ART OF THE SALAD

Salad doesn't have to be token greenery, bland, and perfunctory. In fact, it doesn't even have to be what we think of as salad. You can serve light and nutritious sun-cooked vegetables as:

Crudités. Carrots, celery, bell pepper, zucchini, broccoli, cauliflower, jicama, cucumber, kohlrabi, mushrooms, even thinly sliced turnips, alone or with dip (and with a beginner's book on garnishing and a few simple tools, you can make edible artworks from raw vegies);

Sandwich fillers. Stuffing a pita, rolled in a tortilla, or between slices of bread (salad sandwiches are standard fare in Britain—to be very, very English, use cucumber or watercress);

One-dish meals. By adding cooked beans (try garbanzos or spiced chili beans), brown rice, steamed new potatoes, curly pasta or elbow macaroni, or tofu cubes (marinate them in three parts water to two parts natural tamari soy sauce); have bread or rolls on the side if you wish.

There's an art to the traditional tossed salad as well. You can experiment on your own or use recipes from the recommended cookbooks, but here are general guidelines for a salad you'll actually want to eat.

Choose vegetables for your salad by what's in season, or which imported produce looks fresh and appetizing; and how the colors, textures, and flavors complement each other. Visualize a salad made from iceberg lettuce, peeled cucumber, cauliflower, and mushrooms. Pretty awful, right? There's no color there, no appeal. Now think of that head lettuce with bright red tomato wedges; the cucumber crinkle-cut with its green edge intact; cauliflower set off by grated carrot and a few ripe olives; the mushrooms tossed into a bowl of spinach as green as a St. Patrick's Day hat. Now that's better.

Wash the vegetables you've chosen, giving particular attention to leafy ones like spinach and arugula that collect sediment in their crevices. Dry before putting them in your salad bowl. (A salad spinner does the drying quickly and is fun to use. See "Good Food Gadgets.")

If you use a wooden salad bowl, rub its interior surface with a cut garlic clove. It will impart a wonderful flavor to your salad.

Go easy on oil. The main purpose of using oil in salad is to help herbs and seasonings cling to the vegetables. A tablespoon in a very large salad is sufficient for that. Spraying on oil from a pump bottle instead of pouring it on is an oil-sparing trick. You can actually do without oil altogether if you toss your greens with the juice of a lemon or lime, sprinkle amply with salt-free seasonings (herbal blends like McCormick's Parsley Patch can do wonders for salads), and (optionally) a seasoned salt like Spike. Using cut tomato slices also provides liquid for this "no dressing dressing." Avocado is another useful addition. A rich relative, it is high in oil content but it comes packed with the vitamins, minerals, and fiber of a natural food, something bottled oils can't claim. Even used moderately, avocado can give more satiety value to a salad than oily dressing does, without the use of extracted oils. (Also try topping a plain tossed salad with whatever else is on the menu, like vegetarian chili or baked beans.)

You can dress up a salad with yummy garnishes such as steamed vegetables (asparagus, string beans, broccoli) and small quantities of tasty rich relatives like sunflower seeds and olives.

Make it easy to eat salad. Keep vegetables washed and ready in your fridge at all times. Salad tastes the best when you eat it right after you put it together, but if you need to, make your lunch salad after breakfast and keep it in a large, airtight bowl until noontime. (If you're using dressing, add it right before you eat.)

And remember fresh fruit salads, too. Keep them simple—a melon salad of cubed cantaloupe, honeydew, and casaba melon; a tropical salad of pineapple, tangerine slices, and banana; an autumn salad of apples, grapes, and pears. If you use apple or banana, add a squeeze of lemon to keep their colors true. Make a meal of a fruit salad with the addition of a cashew cream (one-eighth cup raw cashew pieces to four ounces fresh orange juice, blended until smooth) and a sprinkling *of sunflower seeds, raisins, or chopped dates. (A lower fat creamy topping is Banana Milk, included in the recipes in Appendix B. To make Banana Cream, use a little less water.)*

◀ SPROUT FARMING ▶

You don't need a back forty or even a back yard to grow some organic produce of your own. That's because sprout farming can be done anywhere. Even if you skip the alfalfa sprouts on salad bars and can take or leave the mung bean sprouts in Chinese food, you're apt to become much fonder of these "baby vegetables" if you grow them yourself.

Sprouts are seeds that have just begun to germinate, and these tiny plants are bursting with enzymes, vitamins, and minerals while they're shy on calories. Start with good organic seeds (get edible seeds and beans from the health food store, not chemically treated seeds meant for gardening) and count on getting a bundle—at least five pounds—of sprouts from every pound of seed. Among the sprouts you can easily grow are:

Alfalfa
Use raw in salads. These sprout in two to five days.

Dried whole pea
Surprisingly sweet and crunchy, give these two to three days to be ready for salads, snacking, steaming.

Lentil
They take two to three days to sprout and are good raw or cooked; use them in soups and stir-fries.

Peanut
My all-time favorite, peanut sprouts, like other sprouts, are low in fat since the sprouting process requires energy and gets it from the oil present in the unsprouted seed. These are ready in two days, no more than three. (Only raw peanuts will sprout.)

Radish
Spicy! These will perk up an uneventful salad any day. Give them three to five days growing time.

Sunflower seed
These sprout almost as deliciously as peanuts. They are leafy and crunchy at the same time—excellent in salads or on sandwiches.

(You can also grow mung bean sprouts in two to four days, but since you may find it tedious to remove the bitter hulls, you may prefer to purchase these already sprouted. Wheat and other whole grains sprout, too. They can be cooked when barely germinated (after the night's soaking and one day's sprouting time), or used raw as a strangely sweet sprout when allowed to grow four or five days. Soy beans are nearly impossible to sprout at home, but the soy sprouts you can buy at Oriental markets are tasty and substantial. These cannot be eaten raw. Stir-fry them.)

To grow a sprout garden, all you'll need are a Mason jar (a used peanut butter jar will do, or something as large as the institutional-sized food jars you can get from a restaurant or school, if you want a lot of sprouts); a piece of cheesecloth; and a rubber band.[17] Then:

1. Soak seeds (one kind or, if their sprouting times are similar, a variety) in your jar six hours to overnight in pure water. (It's important to use distilled or spring water for this purpose since chlorinated water can impair sprouting.)

2. Cover with cheesecloth cut to go over the top of the jar and attach with rubber band. Drain seeds and rinse them with fresh water (tap water should be okay for the rinsing). You'll want the seeds damp, not wet.

3. Turn the jar on its side at the edge of a sink or in a dish drainer. Rinse and drain two or three times a day until you're ready to harvest. (It's also a good idea to grow your sprouts in the dark—in a cupboard or beneath a dish towel—until the last day when you'll

---

17. There are fancier sprout-growing apparatus of all sorts. You can get some of these at your natural food store. For information on a large variety of equipment, books, and seeds to sprout, contact Sprout House, 40 Railroad St., Great Barrington, MA 01230. A comprehensive book on sprouting, written in a most inviting style, is *SproutGarden: Gourmet Grower's Guide to Sprouts*, by Mark Mathew Braunstein (Ashland, OR: Sprouting Publications, 1992).

*put them in a sunny window to develop chlorophyll and nice green
leaves.)*

As you might imagine, children love to grow sprouts. Sometimes
they'll even eat them.

- - - - - - - - - - - - - - - -

◀ A STEAMY ROMANCE—WITH VEGETABLES! ▶

*Steamed vegetables taste marvelous and take no talent on the cook's
part. Steaming is also the most nutrient-saving cooking method. The
only special equipment required is a stainless steel steaming trivet
available in any cookware department for just a few dollars. To
steam, simply place washed vegetables, whole or cut, in the basket
over boiling water. Make sure the water doesn't touch the vegetables.
Cover tightly and steam until the vegetables are bright and tender-
crisp. When preparing vegetables that require longer cooking, check
the water level and add more water if it's boiling away. Here are
steaming times for some popular vegies:*

Vegetable	Time, in minutes
Beets, medium	*30–40*
Beet greens	*5–6*
Broccoli	*10–15*
Brussels sprouts	*10–15*
Butternut squash	*20–30*
Cabbage	*10–20*
Carrots (sliced)	*10–15*
Carrots (whole)	*20–30*
Collard greens	*8–12*
Green peas, pea pods	*5–10*
Kale	*5–10*
String beans	*12–15*
Sweet potatoes (small to medium, whole, or large, cut)	*25–30*

White potatoes (small to medium, whole, or large, cut)	25–30
Zucchini	10–15

Stir-frying is another cooking method that's quick, easy, and produces a nutritious result. Unlike deep-frying, this technique does not require a large amount of oil. Less than a tablespoon should be enough in a heavy skillet, nonstick pan, or wok. Spread the oil over the surface of the pan and cook quickly, adding other liquids—water, sherry (or optionally apple juice), tomato juice, sodium-reduced tamari—and cook quickly, stirring constantly. If you add extra water and cover intermittently, you're steam-frying, which is a good way to get maximum flavor with minimum fat.

- - - - - - - - - - - - - - - - - -

◄§ SOUP STOCK §►

An organization that wanted a vegetarian luncheon for a seminar was told by a hotel chef, "You cannot make soup without chicken broth!" They changed hotels and got terrific soup. You can make terrific soup, too. Frankly, a perfectly adequate one can be made just starting with water as a base and using miso or tamari (these flavorful soy products are described in the "Natural Foods Glossary" section of this chapter on page 179) for seasoning, or a powdered vegetable broth mix or bouillon. These are available at health food stores. Brands include Vogue Vege Base and Jensen's Broth and Seasoning. Some of the powdered stocks actually taste like chicken or beef if you're looking for that familiar flavor.

If you want to take the homemade route, you can make a stock as good as your grandmother's by following this recipe:

1. Save vegetable scraps and the water left from steaming vegetables. With the exception of cabbage family members (broccoli, cauliflower, etc.) any vegies will do. Clean potato peelings are really good; so are the ends of beans and the tips of carrots. You can use onions, garlic, and mushrooms, too.

2. Add your scraps (and any other vegetables you're using) to

boiling water—about two cups of vegetables to four cups of water. Add some salt, but no more than half a teaspoon.

3. Cover the pot and let the stock simmer just below the boiling point for sixty minutes or so.

4. Let it cool. Strain and discard the vegetables.

Your stock will last in the fridge for a week, or you can freeze it in ice-cube trays. Use it as a base for all kinds of soups—corn chowder, garden vegetable, lentil, minestrone, navy bean, split pea, or potato. You can make cream soups by using soy milk, sesame tahini, blended raw cashews, or even by blending portions of a noncream soup (fresh pea or vegetable), adding a thickener such as arrowroot or cornstarch, and reheating. The cookbooks in Appendix B all have wonderful, easy soup recipes. Soups are one of the best reasons for having winter; and cold soups—gazpacho, fruit soups, and the like—are perfect when it's hot.

If a soup without meat broth, a ham bone, or some other meat seasoning seems like culinary blasphemy, you may want to take the following suggestion. It's from Alvenia Fulton, a traditional naturopath who has an enviable association with Mother Nature and more energy than people half her age. She recommends seasoning stews, casseroles, beans, and vegetables as well as soups with onion, celery, green pepper, and garlic sautéed in vegetable oil. Use one cup of each of the vegies, garlic to taste. Keep this in a covered jar in the refrigerator to take out and use as you need to, the way people used to keep bacon drippings on the back of the stove. Who says you can't start a new tradition?

◄ THE PERFECT POTATO (AND TOPPERS) ►

To bake the perfect potato (or a darn good one at least), choose firm russet potatoes and cut out any "eyes." Prick the skins several times with a fork and bake in a baking dish (this seems to be the secret) in an oven preheated to 450° F. Baking will take about an hour, depending on the size of the potatoes. If you plan to stuff them with other vegetables, they should be fairly large. You can lightly oil the skins if you want to, but don't wrap your potatoes in aluminum foil. There is some evidence that cooking in foil and with aluminum cookware can cause aluminum to build up in the body. This has been theoretically linked with Alzheimer's disease.

The perfect potato deserves the proper topper. Butter is an animal product and, for all intents and purposes, straight, saturated fat. Regular margarine, although made from polyunsaturated oils, has the same fat content as butter, 100%. Diet margarine, although hydrogenated, has half the fat of ordinary margarine or butter. To make any margarine, however, oil is partially hydrogenated to make it solid at room temperature. Hydrogenation creates trans-fatty acids which behave in the body like cholesterol-elevating saturated fat. I admit to using a little margarine on baked potatoes sometimes, but the following toppings, although unorthodox, can be every bit as good.[18]

- Salsa. *Homemade or from a jar*

- Broccoli. *Oversteamed so you can mash it (broccoli stems left after you've cooked the flowerets work just fine), with plenty of freshly ground pepper added*

- Cauliflower. *Just like broccoli*

- Mashed sweet potato or yam. *No kidding; cold leftovers work just fine—sort of like cold butter on a hot potato*

- Carrot butter. *See "Fat Zappers" in this section*

- Tofu spreads. *Try the tofu mayonnaise (with plenty of chives!) in "Tofu 101" in this section*

- Pasta sauce. *With plenty of garlic and basil*

- Barbecue sauce. *Those at health food stores have no refined sugar*

- Gravy. *"White Dill Sauce" from Appendix B, or other lowfat, vegetarian gravies and sauces in the recommended cookbooks*

- Steak sauce. *At restaurants, steak sauce or mustard is sometimes the best you can do, but they're really not bad*

18. Thanks go to Patti Breitman, my literary agent, for several of these ideas.

- Ratatouille. *Sautéed vegetables with tomato sauce, my favorite tater topper*
- Avocado. *"Green butter" mashed or thinly sliced, or seasoned as guacamole*

Use other seasonings—Mrs. Dash, Spike, powdered vegetable broth, scallions, chives—with these toppings and find your own specialties. A potato is fairly dry and mild-tasting, so you're looking for something to provide a little moistness and a touch of spice. Use your imagination!

◀ SANDWICH IDEAS ▶

Every once in a while, you'll still see on a menu the archaic diet plate of cottage cheese, a canned peach half, and a burger without a bun. It would be better to have a bun without a burger! A Love-powered sandwich can, however, be well-filled and come with the bun or both pieces of bread. There are, in fact, a variety of breads to choose from:

- *Whole wheat or whole rye bread, or a gluten-free specialty bread if you're sensitive to wheat*
- *A whole grain pita pocket*
- *A whole wheat English muffin, burger bun, bagel or Kaiser roll*
- *Tortillas, whole wheat or corn*
- *Other unleavened breads—matzoh, chapati, Ethiopian injera*
- *Large crackers—rice cakes, Scottish oatcakes, or Norwegian rye crispbread sold in large rounds to break into right-sized pieces*

Once you've found the bread, you need to fill, top, or spread it. There are dozens of ways to do this. You'll recognize several of the following as rich relatives, so don't overdo the quantities of high-fat or very sweet sandwich fillers. With a good bread and plenty of lettuce and sprouts giving body to a sandwich, you won't have to load on the richer items. Here are some ideas with which to start:

Hummus. *The classic Mideastern spread (or dip) of pureed garbanzo beans and tahini (sesame butter). To keep fat content low, pureed garbanzos by themselves make a good spread. If you use canned ones, drain off all the water except what you'll need to get the blender to run so your spread won't be too thin. Serve hummus or garbanzo puree in pita pockets with plenty of crisp, colorful vegetables.*

Split pea spread. *Leftover split pea soup or cooked split peas thicken in the fridge overnight for a fine sandwich spread. Add more seasonings if you like. This is especially good on hot toast—it almost melts.*

Tofu spreads. *Tofu mayonnaise (see "Tofu 101" in this section) and "Tofu Egg Salad" (the recipe is in Appendix B) make excellent sandwich fillers, with lettuce or sprouts. Marinated tofu slices, heated or not, work well in sandwiches, too. Marinate in two parts water and one part natural tamari soy sauce, season with onion, garlic, even Tabasco® if you're up for it.*

Vegetables. *Thinly sliced cucumber, grated carrot, alfalfa and radish sprouts, lettuce, and sliced tomato are great as stand-alone sandwiches. Try a V.L.T. (vegies, lettuce, and tomato) on a bun with a thin layer of tofu mayonnaise or Dijon mustard, or roll in a tortilla or jchapatti (you can use some steamed vegetables, too).*

Tempeh. *Tempeh makes a meaty sandwich, something like a pork tenderloin but lower in fat and nobody died for it. Readymade tempeh burgers and cutlets (some only need to be heated a minute in a toaster-oven) are in the freezer case at natural food stores. Tempeh generously doused with barbecue sauce at the end of cooking and rolled in a tortilla burrito-style got rave reviews when a firefighter friend of mine fixed it at the firehouse—hardly a bastion of vegetarianism. (For more on tempeh, see* The Book of Tempeh *by William Shurtleff and Akiko Aoyagi, New York: Harper and Row, 1985.)*

Fruit spreads. *Remember jelly sandwiches from childhood? You can make them again using the fruit-only jams and conserves available at both natural food and grocery stores; or you can mix a dried fruit spread by gently simmering for one hour: four cups of chopped dried fruit (a mixture of prunes, raisins, dates, etc.), one-third cup* grated carrots, one-half teaspoon salt, one-third cup lemon juice, one and one-half cups water. Puree in your food processor (metal blade); and simmer again until it thickens.

Avocado. Make into guacamole (mash avocado with chopped tomato and onion, garlic, and chili powder, salt to taste, and a squeeze of lemon to keep avocado from turning brown); or slice thinly and combine with hot mustard, tomato, and sprouts.

Leftovers. Use the vegetarian loaves and burgers you've made for dinner. All the cookbooks listed in Appendix B have recipes for loaves and burgers, usually made from a grain like rice or oats with beans or chopped nuts, vegetables, and seasonings. Some of these can be mashed as is for next day sandwiches. Others mix well with tofu mayonnaise. (Readymade eggless mayonnaise is also available at health food shops. Check the labels; some are as high in fat as conventional mayo, while others are fat-reduced. If you like mustard, it can sometimes substitute for mayo, too.)

Nutbutters. Almond is my favorite. You can cut the fat content of any nutbutter by mixing a tablespoon of it with two tablespoons of water and beating with a fork to emulsify them. You end up with more butter for the same amount of fat. Use nutbutter on one slice of bread, fruit spread on the other. Lettuce and shredded carrots provide a welcome, moist contrast to the dryness of nutbutter and bread. Sliced banana is really good, too. Serve sandwiches with a lot of raw vegetables, a bowl of soup if you like, and an apple later if you're not quite satisfied. This is an ample and easy lunch—and when you bring it to work, I guarantee no one will say, "You must be on another diet."

◀ BEAN CUISINE ▶

Whether we don't know beans about something, or it doesn't amount to a hill of them, beans are disparaged in metaphor and fact. Actually, this staple food comes in more than fifty varieties and has a 9,000-year history of cultivation that has made it important in nourishing and sustaining the human race. Legumes are also a top choice food for the twenty-first century because they're full of fiber and minerals, provide quality protein without the drawbacks of protein from animal sources, and are in most cases very low in fat. They also keep well and are inexpensive. (Beans are cheap enough when you buy them, but when you consider that they swell with water during soaking and cooking, you're getting more satiety for the money. That's the opposite of meat which shrinks when it's cooked, leaving you with less to eat than what you paid for. "You soak beans," said the most frugal cook I know. "They don't soak you.")

To cook beans, presoak them first (with the exception of the smaller legumes, lentils, and split peas, which needn't be soaked). Place them in a large pot with two or three times their volume of water and let them stand for eight hours or overnight. Or to use the quick-soak method, bring the pot to a boil and cook for one minute; turn off the heat, cover the pot, and allow the beans to stand for one to two hours. (The second method is supposed to reduce the likelihood that the beans will cause flatulence. Either way, discard the soaking water and cook in fresh water. The water in which beans are soaked contains sugars that can cause digestive distress.) When you're ready to cook, bring the beans to a boil, then reduce the heat so you can cover the pot and let the beans simmer gently for the indicated amount of time.

Beans can also be pressure-cooked and then do not require a pre-soak. Simply place them in the pressure cooker (three parts water to one part beans). Fill cooker two-thirds full or less. Add one tablespoon oil to prevent foaming. Cover and bring to pressure. Begin timing when gauge rocks. After time is up, cool cooker until pressure is down before removing lid.

The following cooking times are for soaked beans (stove top) and unsoaked (pressure cooker):

	Stove Top	Pressure Cooker
Black beans (turtle beans— small, excellent over rice and in soup)	1½–2 hours	22–25 minutes
Black-eyed peas (Southern tradition says eating these New Year's Day will bring a year's good luck)	1–1½ hours	20 minutes

	Stove Top	Pressure Cooker
Fava beans (broad beans—strong flavor, used in Italian and Middle Eastern cooking)	2–3 hours	40 minutes
Garbanzos (chickpeas—round, golden, flavorful—good in salads and pureed for the dip and spread hummus)	2–3 hours	40 minutes
Great northern beans (white ovals, mild flavor)	1½–2 hours	25 minutes
Kidney beans (the name tells the shape of these dark red beans with a meaty taste and mealy texture)	1½–2 hours	30 minutes
Lentils (Small, flat red or brown-green pulses, wonderful in soups, loaves)	30 minutes	Don't pressure-cook
Lima beans (colored creamy to light green, these mild beans come in large and small varieties)	Small: 1–1½ hours Large: 2 hours	20 minutes 30 minutes
Navy beans (little white ovals, nice in soups and stews)	2 hours	30 minutes
Pinto beans (the Latin specialty so good in chili and dips—"refry" without oil by simply blending cooked, seasoned pintos in a blender)	1½–2 hours	25 minutes
Soybeans (pea-sized beans usually light yellow; products made from them—tofu, tempeh, etc.—are easier to use and therefore more popular)	2½–3 hours	30–35 minutes

	Stove Top	Pressure Cooker
Split peas (green or yellow, cook fairly quickly, good with rice, for soups; leftovers can be turned into a sandwich spread)	*30 minutes*	*Don't pressure-cook*

◄§ TOFU 101 §►

Do you have some friends that you really had to get to know before you liked them? Tofu is like that. Once you get friendly with it, the odds are good you'll be glad you did. Tasteless on its own, tofu can take on flavorings used with it to become a worthy pinch hitter for such diverse—and cholesterol-laden—foods as ground beef, chicken, mayonnaise, cream cheese, sour cream, and even eggs.

Made from soybeans, the richest in oil of all legumes, tofu weighs in at 53% fat per calorie. It's not a lowfat food when compared with other Love-powered choices like bananas (3%), cabbage (7%), and kidney beans (4%). But filling in for cream cheese (91% fat), hamburger (65%), or eggs (65%) there is a savings—not to mention that switching to tofu eliminates the other problems that come with using animal foods. Tofu is economical, easy to digest, and (if precipitated with calcium sulfate), a good source of calcium. If you miss animal foods, if you have a family to cook for that's resistant to change, or if you entertain a lot, tofu can make things easier.

So let's get acquainted! By itself, tofu is like wet foam rubber, but you'd no more eat it by itself and expect fine dining than you'd stare at a blank canvas and expect fine art. To become a Rembrandt with tofu, you first need to:

1. Find it—Tofu is usually in the produce department with the Oriental vegetables. If you don't find it there, look in the dairy case where it's sometimes kept because it's so easily interchangeable with cottage, pot, farmer, feta, or ricotta cheese. You can also locate tofu in aseptic packages so that it needs no refrigeration, or environmentally unpackaged *for bulk sale at natural food stores and Oriental markets.*

2. *Select it—Tofu is often labeled according to its consistency: extra firm, firm, soft, and silken (very soft). Firm can be used for everything; soft for dips, sauces, and spreads. The extremes (extra firm and silken) are less versatile.*

3. *Store it—Tofu must be kept in water. If you get it in bulk, store it in bowls of water in your refrigerator. If it comes in a nonsealed carton (like cottage cheese), put in fresh water when you get it home and refrigerate it that way. If your tofu is vacuum-packed, put fresh water on any leftovers after it's been opened. Change the water every two or three days. Fresh tofu so cared for will last a week to ten days in the fridge.*[19] *(Vacuum-packed tofu lasts quite a while when refrigerated; check the date on the container before you buy.)*

All the cookbooks recommended in Appendix B have some recipes using tofu. If you want to go even further, I recommend Tofu Cookery by Louise Hagler (Summertown, TN: The Book Publishing Co., rev. ed., 1991), a classic cookbook revised to feature simplified and lower fat recipes; and The Book of Tofu by William Shurtleff and Akiko Aoyagi (Berkeley, CA: Ten Speed Press, rev. ed., 1983), the volume that introduced this multifaceted food to the West. For easy fixin's, start with these:

Salad dressing. *Add to tofu in blender a bit of lemon juice or cider vinegar, tamari (natural soy sauce), water as needed for the consistency you want, and whatever seasonings you fancy. My favorite is dried dill weed, and garlic and onion powder are always good. So is the spicy combo curry and cumin.*

Tofu mayonnaise. *Drain tofu. Place in blender or food processor a 6-ounce chunk along with 2 tablespoons of lemon juice, 1 tablespoon oil, ½ teaspoon salt, ¼ teaspoon white pepper, and puree. Add sea-*

---

19. It is possible to freeze tofu. Standard procedure is to press out all its water, crumble the tofu, and freeze for "ground tofu" to use like ground beef in chili and sloppy joes. The freezing process changes the consistency of tofu entirely. The result is a spongy product that some people believe tastes more like meat. Personally, I think freezing ruins perfectly decent tofu. Give it a try and see what you think.

sonings if you want—onion, garlic, pickle, etc. (To lower fat content, omit the oil.)

Sandwich spreads. Mix mashed tofu with chopped vegetables like carrots and celery. Thin with tofu mayo to spreading consistency.

Burgers. Mix mashed tofu with chopped or grated vegies (onions, bell pepper, mushrooms, or your choice) and some sesame or ground sunflower seeds. Use flour to make mixture stiff enough to form burgers. Season with salt, tamari, basil, cumin, garlic, onion, whatever. Bake or broil.

Tofu loaf. Use mashed tofu instead of ground beef in a meatloaf recipe.

Tofu steaks. Drain tofu. Slice in half-inch thicknesses. Coat with flour and spices. Bake till they're crisp. (This is extra good if you marinate the tofu first in half water, half tamari.)

Soup. Cut drained tofu in little squares and use to replace chicken in chicken soup. Use a chicken-flavored vegetarian broth mix from the health food store for the base. Simmer long enough for tofu to pick up the flavor.

Pudding or "yogurt". Puree in food processor tofu, sweetener (maple syrup is nice), vanilla, and a dash of salt. Adding carob powder makes a "chocolate" pudding. (If you're a real yogurt fan, cultured soy yogurt is sold readymade at many natural food stores. If you make yogurt yourself, that can be done with soy milk, too. There is a recipe for it in Ten Talents, one of the cookbooks in Appendix B.)

◄ THE GRANARY ►

Solid, centering whole grains are the staples of a Love-powered diet. Although they're filling and filled with a wide range of minerals and B vitamins, a full cup averages less than two grams of fat.

Most grains can be:

Cooked. *For (a) a hot breakfast cereal (use extra water if you won't be topping with soy or nut milk; cook with dried fruit for a sweetener, perhaps overnight in a crock-pot, or sweeten with a little maple syrup or date sugar); (b) a side dish (i.e., rice to make a bed for black beans or stir-fried vegetables); or (c) an entrée (rice pilaf, millet stuffing for squash or peppers, couscous served with steamed vegetables)*

Sprouted. *Wheat and rye sprout particularly well*

Ground into flour. *Whole wheat flour for yeast breads, whole wheat pastry flour for quick breads, cookies, pie crusts; corn meal for corn bread, muffins, and Johnny cakes; buckwheat for pancakes; brown rice, millet, and rye flours for specialty baking or as alternatives to wheat for people with allergies*

Made into pasta. *Whole wheat spaghetti and lasagne noodles are found in supermarkets; health food stores not only stock these, but also pastas made from corn, rice, and buckwheat*

Whole grains can also be used in soups (barley is a natural here), in salads (rice, pasta), or in desserts like rice or bread pudding. Rice is even made into a sweet, nourishing drink (amasake), a liquid sweetener (rice syrup), and an ice cream-like frozen dessert[20] (the brand name is Rice Dream®).

Your supermarket can provide you with whole wheat bread (be sure the wrapper says one hundred percent whole wheat), whole wheat pasta, brown rice, brown rice pilaf (one brand name is Near East), wild rice, oatmeal, and whole grain cold cereals like Nutri-Grain and shredded wheat. Health food stores have a vast array of whole grains as well as the flours, pastas, and cereals made from them. There are exotic grains to try like sticky-sweet amaranth and light, fluffy quinoa. And there are the basics:

---

20. Several nondairy frozen desserts are on the market. Any sorbet or "ice" is nondairy, and among those that replicate ice cream convincingly are Ice Bean® and Believe®, both soy-based. These desserts are designed to take the place of ice cream, so an ice cream addict would need to be alert to a possible binge food potential with these. Because they are lower in fat than ice cream and contain no refined sugar, most people can enjoy them without a problem.

Brown rice. *Long-grain brown rice cooks up in separate kernels to eat as is or use in pilafs; short-grain turns out sticky, good for croquettes and burgers or even pressed onto a pie plate as a fat-free crust for a tofu quiche or vegetable pie. Basmati is a gourmet rice from India with a nutty flavor and wonderful aroma. You can buy both brown and white Basmati rice.*

Buckwheat (kasha). *Cook this like rice or as a hot breakfast cereal. Buckwheat flour is fabulous for hotcakes.*

Millet. *Tiny round grains that become puffy and delicate when cooked, millet can be used as a cooked cereal, stuffing, the base for burgers, or as a side dish.*

Oats. *You can cook whole oats (called groats), but oatmeal—even the quick-cooking kind—is a whole grain, too. Use for breakfast, in baking, or as the base for vegie-burgers. (You can eat extracted oat bran if you want, but you may as well get the bran with the rest of the oat as a whole food.)*

Scotch barley. *This is whole grain barley; the refined kind is called pearl barley. Use in soups or as an alternative to rice.*

Whole wheat. *Whole wheat berries may be cooked or sprouted as well as ground into flour for bread or pasta. Couscous is a quick-cooking wheat product that has been presteamed. Most of the couscous available is refined, but even if you can't find the whole grain variety, this quick-cooking, company-pleasing grain can have a place in your Love-powered pantry.*

Bulgur. *Bulgur is cracked wheat, popular in Middle Eastern cooking, and the primary ingredient for the wheat salad, tabouli.* Wheat germ *is the nutritious heart of the wheat kernel. It's therefore not a whole (intact) food, and it's rich enough in oil to qualify as a rich relative. However, it is a concentrated source of vegetable protein and vitamin E. When you are not using it, keep wheat germ stored in the fridge. And buy it toasted since raw wheat germ can go rancid very quickly.* Wheat bran *is sold separately, too, for dietary fiber, but the whole grain provides both the bran and the germ.*

Wild rice. *An elegant addition to a special meal, this North American native can dress up an ordinary rice dish or make an exquisite stuffing for winter squash.*

And although we don't tend to think of corn as a grain, we use corn meal as such. Whole corn meal—germ and bran included—is available at natural food stores to use for hot cereal or breads.

All these whole grains keep well. Store them in jars with tightfitting lids, and keep the jars in a cool, dry place. Refrigerate whole grain flours.

When it comes to cooking them, author Nava Atlas offers the simple suggestions of first rinsing the grains in a fine sieve (presteamed, rolled grains such as rolled oats don't require this); optionally, toasting in a dry or lightly oiled skillet until the grains turn a shade darker and release a nutty aroma; boiling the necessary water, stirring in the grain, returning to the boil, lowering the heat, and simmering, covered, until the water is absorbed.

"Do not stir while the grain is cooking. (Note: Rolled oats, bulgur, and couscous do not require simmering; just turn off heat and allow grain to sit for the specified time.) If grains are too chewy for your liking at the end of cooking time, add another one-half cup of water for every cup of raw grain used; cover and simmer until water is absorbed."[21]

Here are the cooking times for some of the grains you'll want to try. These times assume that you're using two parts water to one part grain. Until you're used to whole grains, listen a little ahead of time to see if the simmering sound has stopped so you don't scorch a pot.

Cooking Times for Sample Grains

Brown rice	*45 minutes*
Buckwheat groats (kasha)	*20 minutes*
Bulgur, cracked wheat	*15 minutes*

21. This, as well as some of the grain facts used here, come from "The Essential Guide to Grains" by Nava Atlas, an article which appeared in the August 1989 issue of *Vegetarian Times* magazine. Used with permission of the author. For additional information, see *The Wholefood Catalog* by Nava Atlas (NY: Fawcett-Columbine, 1988).

Millet	40 minutes
Quinoa	15 minutes
Rolled oats	10 minutes
Wheat berries	60–90 minutes

◀ FAT ZAPPERS ▶

Our bodies don't require eggs or dairy foods or extracted oils, but for the kind of cooking we're used to, these foods seem essential. The cookbooks in Appendix B can make you a masterful chef—or as close to that as you care to be—using no animal products and little oil. For now, this conversion chart should suffice. Most of these really zap the fat!

Eggs

Whole eggs, scrambled. *Consult cookbooks for recipes for scrambled tofu, or try the commercial product, Tofu Scrambler, from Fantastic Foods, found at your natural food store.*

In baking. *For each egg use 1 teaspoon commercial egg replacer plus 2 tablespoons water; or 1 tablespoon arrowroot powder, 1 tablespoon soy flour, plus 2 tablespoons water; or 2 tablespoons flour, ½ tablespoon vegetable shortening, ½ teaspoon baking powder, plus 2 tablespoons water; or 2 ounces tofu blended with the liquid called for in the recipe; or ½ large banana, mashed.*

In casseroles, burgers and loaves. *Replace one egg with*[22] *mashed potato; or mashed avocado (high fat, no cholesterol); or moistened breadcrumbs or rolled oats.*

Dairy

Milk. *Commercial soy milk (there are lowfat varieties); powdered soy milk (be sure to get soy milk powder, not soy flour); rice milk,*

---

22. Thanks go to Mariclare Barrett Obis, food editor of *Vegetarian Times*, for these egg replacement tips and for a great deal of the general information on cooking that I put into practice every day and am sharing with you in this section.

"Rice Dream®" and "amasake"; nut milk (almond, cashew, see cookbooks); banana milk (in Appendix B).

Cheese. Mashed soft tofu (for ricotta); soy cheese (in the dairy case at natural food stores. Most contain casein, a milk derivative, but at least one is 100% dairy-free. One of those containing casein is marketed as fat-free. The others have a fat content comparable to that of dairy cheese but with no cholesterol); small amounts of miso or tamari to add salty flavor; nutritional yeast or the rich relative tahini (sesame butter) can substitute for parmesan on pasta; for cream cheese, use firm tofu blended with salt, dill, and lime juice to taste.

Butter. In addition to margarine and oil, which should only be used very moderately, try nutbutters (high in fat but nourishing and natural), fruit spreads, and Mary McDougall's Carrot Butter[23]:

CARROT BUTTER

4 medium-size carrots, scrubbed and finely chopped or grated
½ cup water
1½ tablespoons carrot-cooking liquid
2 tablespoons natural peanut butter
1 tablespoon frozen orange juice concentrate

Put the carrots and water in a small saucepan and bring to a boil. Cover, lower the heat, and simmer for ½ hour, stirring occasionally. Drain the carrots and reserve the liquid. Place the carrots, 1½ tablespoons cooking liquid, peanut butter, and orange juice concentrate in the blender and process until very smooth, stopping blender and stirring contents as needed. Add more liquid only if absolutely necessary, as the mixture should be thick. Chill thoroughly (as least 1 hour) before using.

Use as a substitute for butter on cooked vegetables, and potatoes or as a spread for muffins. It keeps well in the refrigerator.

Makes about 1 cup
Preparation Time: 15 min. plus 1 hour chilling time; Cooking Time: 30 min.

23. From The McDougall Program: Twelve Days to Dynamic Health, by John Mc-Dougall, M.D., with recipes by Mary McDougall. This is among the listings in Appendix A. The McDougall Program's recipes also include instructions for making "cheese" (with the grain millet), cheesy sauces, and spreads.

Oils

In baking. *Substitute natural applesauce for the oil or butter you would otherwise use (another trick from Mary McDougall).*

On vegetables. *Marilyn Diamond's Oil-Free Herb Sauce (see Appendix B).*

Salad dressings. *Blend vegetables and herbs with tomato and lemon juice; see oil-free salad dressing recipes in Appendix B; cut oil in conventional recipes by half and substitute tomato juice or blended tofu; blend a small amount of nuts, seeds, or avocado (all high-fat but non-fragmented) with carrot, celery or tomato juice, or with water, lemon, and savory seasonings to taste; squeeze fresh lime on a salad to allow the taste of the vegetables to come through—fresh lime or lemon and a seasoned salt or herbal blend make for a sophisticated salad.*

For stove top cooking. *Use nonstick cookware to eliminate or cut down on oil (high quality cookware with tight-fitting lids retains steam from vegetables, minimizing the amount of oil and other liquid required);*

Coat pans with liquid lecithin instead of oil (the lecithin sprays work, too, but please avoid any aerosol products with CFC propellants that destroy the ozone);

Use other liquids for cooking besides oil: water, tomato juice, cooking sherry or apple juice, tamari (soy sauce—the sodium-reduced kind works best for cooking), vegetable broth, or an oil/water combination (try 1 tablespoon oil to ⅓ cup water).

◀ GOOD FOOD GADGETS ▶

You won't need a kitchen filled with paraphernalia to create Love-powered meals your body will truly appreciate. The important utensils will be some nice wooden spoons for stirring, a big bowl or two for mixing and for salads, some sharp paring knives, a couple of pieces of good, nonaluminum cookware with lids, a vegetable steamer, and either a blender or a food processor for making spreads, sauces, smoothies, cream soups, and the like.

Among the following good food gadgets, you'll find some you already own and some you may want to invest in. Skip the others, or give them as wedding presents.

Blender. *Ideal for shakes and smoothies, also for making nut milk.*

Champion Juicer. *I mention a brand name only because this is the one machine I'm familiar with that can make the soft-serve, fruit-based frozen desserts mentioned in Chapter 8 in our discussion of bananas and mangoes. The Champion also juices vegetables and fruits and makes fresh nutbutters. It is sold in natural food stores.*

Citrus Juicer. *Inexpensive models, either manual or electric, are found in discount, department, and cookware stores. Fresh grapefruit, orange, and tangerine juices are exquisite!*

Double Boiler. *Two pots, one holds boiling water. Cooks gently, excellent for preparing grains such as millet or for reheating leftovers.*

Food Processor. *Shreds, chops, mixes, and kneads. Helpful for making salads, dips, and purees.*

Hot Air Popcorn Popper. *For fat-free popcorn that you can season yourself with tamari, nutritional yeast (for a cheesy taste), or a dash of cayenne.*

Mortar and Pestle. *Spices are best when freshly ground and this is the time-honored way to do it. (An electric coffee and spice mill is another option.)*

Nonstick Cookware. *Cut down on oil use by investing in at least one high quality, nonstick pan. Get a good one with a lengthy guarantee against chipping of the coating. It's also sensible to look for nonstick cookware that doesn't require the use of special utensils: unless you live alone, someone is bound to use the wrong spatula at some point. (I don't believe that all cookware needs to be nonstick. Have at least one piece—a Dutch oven or soup pot perhaps—in cast iron to maximize the iron in your diet.)*

Pressure Cooker. *Popular in the 1950s, pressure cookers are back in more sophisticated models. Pressure-cooking is a real time saver when beans are on the menu.*

Salad Spinner. *This nifty contraption in cookware departments and gourmet shops will spin-dry salad greens in a jiffy.*

Slow Cooker. *Let a slow cooker (crockpot) simmer up a one-pot dinner (soup, stew, chili, homemade grain pilaf) while you're gone all day. (Mary McDougall's cookbooks are an excellent resource for slow cooker recipes. See Appendix B.)*

Sprouter. *If you'd like to grow sprouts in a more sophisticated manner than the cheesecloth and jar technique described earlier, there are perforated plastic trays, special bamboo bags, and a variety of other inventions for growing your sprout garden. Check at your natural foods store.*

Vegetable Juicer. *The Champion is one kind of vegetable juicer. Another type uses centrifugal force for extracting the juice from fruits and vegetables. Health food stores have the best selection, but vegetable juicers are now also available in cookware departments.*

Vegetable Steamer. *You can get yourself vitamins and great taste you would otherwise miss in cooked vegetables by buying a stainless steel vegetable steaming rack for little more than pocket change. Place it over boiling water in a pot with a tight-fitting lid; put the vegetables on top; and say "yummy" a few minutes later.*

Wok. *You can stir-fry in a large skillet, but a wok—an electric wok or one that you put on the stove—invites the frequent use of this healthful style of cooking. Look into a nonstick wok to keep oil use to a minimum.*

You'll notice that I didn't mention microwaves. It's true that they save time and energy, and they can be a real help in cooking without added fats. If you already have one, you probably love it, so use it in good health. I don't recommend microwaves, however, for three reasons. First, I don't trust them yet. Although they appear to be safe, Marilyn Diamond writes, "At present there are over 100 research studies ongoing, funded by the U.S. government, on the safety of mi-

crowave radiation. The question we ought to be asking is, if micro-waves are safe enough to warrant the vast popularity they have achieved, why is so much research still going on?"[24] Regular monitor-ing for leakage is, at least, an important precaution.

My second argument with the microwave is that I don't think that microzapped food tastes as good as food cooked conventionally. As a practicing binge eater, I ate food no matter how it tasted. I don't have to do that today. Today I can have the best, even if it means waiting for it.

Third, I think too much dependence on microwaving—as well as on fast-food restaurants—can impede a food addict's recovery. Both quickly provide food that can be quickly eaten, which is the ideal set-up for a binge. When you cook beans and grains the old-fashioned way, taking your time is a given. When you're eating raw fruits and vegetables, there's no time spent fixing them, but plenty goes into chewing! Either way, a slow-down factor is built in. I have found in my own experience a good deal of value in this.

Also of value is seeing that your kitchen is a place that makes you smile. If yours is filled with unhappy memories of sneaking leftovers and midnight refrigerator raids, christen it as a new place, a friendly place supportive of your true needs and of a Love-powered life. Hang up a picture you treasure or quotations that mean something to you. You may want to treat yourself to new tableware. When I had a set of pottery dishes made that I'd designed myself, I felt special. A bit of that feeling has stayed with each plate and bowl and mug. That makes every meal with these dishes a special occasion, even though the set cost no more than ordinary stoneware.

Start with small things. Delight in your dishes or your herb plants or the needlework saying on the wall. You'll soon delight as well in how your eating has changed. It's all connected.

24. Marilyn Diamond, *American Vegetarian Cooking from the Fit for Life Kitchen*, p. 28.

◀ KITCHEN ECOLOGY ▶

Simply eating Love-powered foods and leaving others behind takes some pressure off the earth. Other simple practices you can undertake as you do your grocery shopping and food preparation can lighten the planet's burden even more. Among these are:

- *Use cloth or string bags when you shop. If you've lived outside North America, you already know this as a natural and pleasant way to shop. If you're without your cloth bags, paper is probably a better choice than plastic. Either way, please reuse and then recycle them.*

- *Buy in bulk when you can. Natural food stores and co-ops often offer whole grains, flours, nuts, seeds, dried fruit, maple syrup, tofu, and other foods in bulk, allowing you to use your own refillable containers.*

- *When you have a choice, choose the product with the least packaging.*

- *Store foods in jars you've saved or in other reusable containers to cut down on your use of plastic wrap and foil. Also you can try cellulose storage bags made from plant fiber.[25]*

- *Save energy by including lots of raw foods in your diet and by not cooking at the highest heat setting.*

- *Compost your food scraps. This actually turns your garbage into rich soil that can be used in a garden or simply donated back to the earth. It's easier than you think. A helpful book is Stu Campbell's* Let It Rot.[26]

- *Forego the disposable chopsticks at Chinese restaurants (or bring your own reusable pair). Disposable chopsticks are taking their toll on bamboo forests.*

25. Your natural food store may carry these. If not, send for the catalog from Seventh Generation, Products for a Healthy Planet, Colchester, VT 05446-1672.
26. Stu Campbell, *Let It Rot! The Home Gardener's Guide to Composting*, (Storey Publications, Pownal, VT, 1990).

- Keep a mug at the office instead of using Styrofoam, and suggest a switch to washable cups to your church, club groups, etc.

- Use cloth napkins. To make this practical, you won't want all your napkins lace-edged or made of heavy linen. Look into the cotton and cotton/poly bandanas reasonably priced at camping equipment stores. One napkin a week per family member may be enough, but keep plenty on hand for guests, spills, and messy meals.

- Avoid the energy drain of your dishwasher's drying cycle by allowing clean dishes to air-dry. And whether you do your dishes by machine or with a pair of rubber gloves, use a detergent that's environmentally sound and cruelty-free (that is, safety-tested without the use of live animals). You can find these at natural food stores and in mail-order catalogs such as those from Seventh Generation (see footnote 25) and The Compassionate Consumer, Box 27, Jerico, NY 11753.

Every concerned and loving action you take shows the Love-empowerment working in your life. Using a cloth bag instead of plastic is like making yourself a couple of baked potatoes instead of tearing into a bag of chips. Both show you care, and it's pretty difficult to practice genuine caring and to practice addiction at the same time.

-✺-

NINE

The

Love-Powered

Life

A Love-powered life is a life of love and power. The power doesn't come from the personal ego—defined, someone recently told me, as "Edging God Out"—but from the unlimited power of Love. When we talk about the power that heats our houses and runs our cars, the synonym we use for it is energy. Adopting Love-powered principles, spiritually and physically, brings abundant energy into our lives. For one thing, there's more energy available from eating this way: unrefined carbohydrates are known for fueling endurance athletes. And we can take advantage of greater energy still because of the changes that have taken place in our thoughts and attitudes. How that energy is spent can define a Love-powered life.

There is nothing dogmatic about this. There are no rules imposed from the outside. You have your own connection with universal Love, a connection to be respected. In general, though, a Love-powered life can be recognized by its ABCs. A Love-powered life is addiction-free, balanced, and compassionate.

Addiction-free. Spiritual renewal makes freedom from addiction possible. Sensible choices on the physical level are supportive of this. Spiritual renewal and sensible choices have been dealt with at length already. With daily rededication to your new way of life, you can expect not only freedom from the food fix but freedom from other imbalances that have held you back.

Balance. True balance comes about when generous portions of love and power (energy) are expressed harmoniously in a person's life. I think of it as working like this:

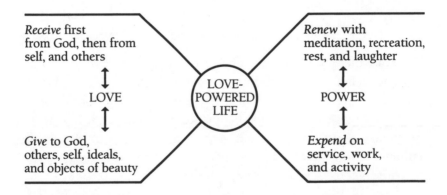

Receive first from God, then from self, and others ↕ LOVE ↕ Give to God, others, self, ideals, and objects of beauty

LOVE-POWERED LIFE

Renew with meditation, recreation, rest, and laughter ↕ POWER ↕ Expend on service, work, and activity

In practice, giving and receiving love become the same thing. Love can't be stored up like grain in a silo or pennies in a jar, so the love you get must go out again. **You become a conduit rather than a container. The more love you give, the more you're able to channel. It's the ultimate in recycling.** Energy operates similarly. You renew your supply in quiet times with your Higher Power, in rest and sleep, and by having fun. You expend it when you work, play, or give service; yet work that you love, exuberant activity, and doing some good in the world give energy back to you, too.

Compassion. Love and energy, giving and receiving, expending and renewing, enable lives to work. Lives that work best also reveal *compassion*. Compassion is the keynote of the eating plan suggested here and compassion, although interpreted in different ways, is central to any viable spirituality. Its literal meaning is "to feel with." You can "feel with" another because you've been hurt yourself and can empathize, or because you've had compassion shown to you and you know how to pass it on. If you are a recovering food addict, you've experienced both—the hurt of the addiction, and then the compassion of your Higher Power, supportive friends, and your own compassion for yourself as you became willing to live without the familiar crutch of excess food.

In this chapter, we'll explore addiction-free, Love-powered living as it

1. Expresses balance: a healthy, harmonious lifestyle; and as it

2. Expresses compassion: "feeling with" others and having love and energy to devote to them

◄ THE BALANCE OF HEALTHFUL LIVING ►

There are many ways in which balance can be evident in a life: harmonious relationships, productive work, responsible financial dealings. Here we'll look at balance in terms of taking good care of ourselves physically since food addiction robs that from its victims most often. As you progress in Love-powered living, you will develop enough self-love to want to care for yourself and enough energy to do it. The self-care, then, creates even more energy.

There are, in any case, some specific laws of life which, when followed, lead to health and happiness. When they're ignored or denied, we get the opposite results. These important laws include:[1]

· Eating pure food that enhances physical well-being

· Taking regular, vigorous exercise

· Getting plenty of rest and sleep

---

1. These are adapted from literature of the American Natural Hygiene Society. (See listing in Appendix C.) *Fit for Life II: Living Health* by Harvey and Marilyn Diamond details these and other natural laws that promote a healthy life. (See Appendix A.)

- Breathing fresh air
- Drinking pure water
- Establishing a respectful relationship with the sun
- Managing stress levels and developing emotional poise

I used to think that if a person were spiritual enough, the physical wouldn't matter. **Today I see "spiritual" and "physical" as concentric circles, or colors in a rainbow, one fading into the next. The fact that there are natural laws to help us get more joy out of life is as close to a gift from God as anything I know of.**

As an active food addict, taking care of myself was near the bottom of my priority list. I can slide back into some of the old ways now, but natural law is there for my benefit—yours, too—all the time. Maybe I didn't get enough sleep last night, or maybe I didn't exercise for five days straight. I can take a nap *now*. I can exercise *today*. So can you. And these healthy habits are self-propagating. Once you make room for them in your life, things don't seem right without them.

Now let's explore each of these laws of life individually. We covered the issue of food choices in Chapters 6, 7, and 8. Here we'll look at the importance of exercise, rest, fresh air, pure water, sunlight, and emotional poise.

Love Yourself with Activity

Exercise is good for the body, but it's even better for the spirit. Well before you observe that an increase in your activity level has blessed you with firmer muscles, greater stamina, and a more efficient metabolic rate, you will notice a heightened sense of well-being and self-worth. I know this is true even though I have a long history of detesting almost any endeavor capable of producing perspiration. In recent years, I've come to appreciate how good moving my body can make me feel. Sometimes I love it. Sometimes I just go through the motions. When I start to truly dislike the exercise I'm doing, I know it's time to change it. That's because the body doesn't exercise alone; the mind comes along, too, and it also needs to enjoy itself.

It's not always easy because even the vocabulary that refers to physical activity makes it seem like chain gang labor. "Exercise" sounds like "exertion." People can be hospitalized for that! A "workout" doesn't sound like a great good time either. My friend Dr. Douglas Graham, surely one of the fittest people I know, tells his patients, "I don't want you to work out. You work all day. In your free time, I expect you to *play*."

Someone who is already fit like Dr. Graham might play as he does—trampolining in his backyard, hiking in the Maine woods, skiing in Colorado, swimming in the Gulf of Mexico, taking 100-mile bike trips, or maneuvering through town on rollerblades with the agility of a carefree school kid on the first day of summer vacation. People who have been battling their bodies for years, however, don't automatically equate exercise with play or pleasure. "Workout" seems like a most appropriate term, because hard exercise taken too soon can feel like work, drudgery even, and for someone with a very low level of fitness, demeaning drudgery.

Most of us who were overweight as children have horrible memories about sports and athletics. We were chosen last for teams, and grudgingly at that. We were called names by our classmates, chided by physical education teachers, and we experienced real suffering doing what everyone else apparently regarded as fun. We rubbed sores on our thighs when we tried to run. Our throats burned as we gasped for air, hoping to keep up in the sprint or make it to the bases. And the emotional pain of being seen in a swimsuit or showering after gym class was as acute as any physical discomfort.

Specific, conscious memories can fade, but those painful feelings attach themselves in our minds to the entire realm of exercise and participatory sports. It's no wonder that even after we're grown up, many of us regard exercise as a threat.

People who were not heavy in childhood but gained extra weight later can have another problem. They remember how good it once felt to run and jump and dance. Thinking that they can't do these things now makes them feel sad and old when decades of promise still lie before them.

SURPRISE! You *can* move your body and you can *enjoy* doing it— now! Whether you were fat as a child or not, and regardless of your current weight or age, you will be a happier as well as a fitter person when you start to use your muscles *regularly* and *pleasurably*. Remember that we're talking about a Love-powered approach to diet and a

Love-powered approach to life. A "no pain, no gain" philosophy does not fit here. *Taking it slow is not only advisable, it is mandatory.*

For exercise to do for you all that it can, it has to become an integral part of your life. It's not to be used, like some willpower diet, just until you get thin. And it's not to be put off until after you're thin, after you save the money to join a health club, or after you get around to putting air in your bicycle tires at some nebulous future point. You do it today because *your body is a living organism that craves movement.* Look at toddlers and puppies; the urge to be active is innate. If you think that urge in you is dead, it isn't. It's only sleeping. Don't try to jolt it awake with fifty pushups and a five-mile run. Nudge it gently.

If you're over forty, overweight, or if you have health problems requiring a special exercise regimen (diabetes, high blood pressure, heart disease, and arthritis are among these), by all means work out your fitness program with a knowledgeable physician. In any case, begin slowly. This is not just because it's easier on your heart and your joints to build up gradually. It's also because if you don't love what you're doing, you're likely to leave it. Sporadic exercise, a week here, a weekend there, a long layoff, then a ski trip, does almost nothing for a body and is an open invitation to injury.

Ideally, Love-powered exercise is what you do because you love yourself *and* the activity. The forms of exercise you choose may change because it is not necessary that you be a distance runner, a belly dancer, or a power lifter. What is necessary for a fit and healthy life is that you be active enough for your body to function optimally. The general rule for accomplishing this is a minimum of twenty minutes of aerobic exercise three times a week. Aerobic (oxygen utilizing) exercises are those that can be done for prolonged periods: walking, running, swimming, skating, cycling, rowing, dancing, etc. This type of exercise is believed to be of particular benefit to the heart and circulatory system, to revive a sluggish metabolism, and to help normalize an unreasonable appetite.

Aerobic activity is not the only sort of useful motion that exists, however. The luxurious limbering and stretching of yoga and modern dance promote youthful flexibility, and strength-building exercises like weight training can sculpt a body to its best and provide it with more lean tissue. Dr. John McDougall writes:

The formation of more muscle tissue is . . . an advantage to a person who wants to lose weight, because the many mitochondria (energy-producing structures) that are found in muscle cells consume considerably greater quantities of fuel than do the few mitochondria in the rather inert fat cells of the body. Thus, your own body will be burning more of the calories you bring into it by eating if you improve the ratio of muscle tissue to fat tissue on your frame. . . . Men and women who go in for exercises that increase strength, like body building, not only get a better-looking body . . . but also get a better functioning one.[2]

If you're approaching, or reapproaching, exercise as a beginner, choose something you think you'll *like* and something you think you'll *do*. If you're a loner, you might want to invest in a stationary bike or a home treadmill. If you love the outdoors, you'll probably prefer to jog or cycle whenever weather permits and schedule some enjoyable backup activity when it doesn't. If you're gregarious, you'll like taking classes or belonging to a gym. Don't expect your basic personality to change to fit some arbitrary exercise plan. It's not about to.

I, for example, live with a state-of-the-art treadmill. Am I using it? Not on your life. I'm at my desk communicating with you. I'm a communicator, one of the gregarious types. When I'm at the health club, I exercise (and communicate!) most energetically; but if I had to exercise at home by myself, I'd probably be suffering from advanced muscle atrophy. However, since exercise is now an expected part of my life, one that I miss when I'm deprived of it, I'd find some sociable exercise even if I couldn't belong to a gym. Maybe I'd invite people in to watch an aerobics video three mornings a week, or join a group that walks at the mall. Whatever it took, I'd get my needs met, both my personality's need for contact with people and my body's need for vigorous physical activity.

Some of the ways you may wish to meet your inborn need for activity are:

Walking. Where do you like to walk? Through the woods? Along country roads? I love to walk in cities. From my point of view, the best part of being in New York or Chicago or San Francisco is walking all

2. John McDougall, M.D., *The McDougall Program: Twelve Days to Dynamic Health*, pp. 70–71. (See Appendix A.)

over, feeding pigeons, snooping in shop windows, exploring parks and cathedrals, and taking in the sounds and sights and energy of the city. When walking is your activity of choice, you can do it anywhere, and the only equipment it takes is a pair of sturdy, well-fitting walking shoes.

If you don't like the idea of exercise, see your walking as simply "taking a walk." My friend Robin calls people she knows and asks if they'd like to walk with her the way we would more often ask someone out for a drink or a meal. It's a really charming invitation. Or walk in your own company. Then you can vary your pace to suit yourself. Your walking may evolve into jogging or race-walking. On alternating days when you aren't looking for a bona fide aerobic workout, you might forego speeding things up in favor of slowing them down. Then you can treat yourself to the serenity of walking meditation. Of this practice Thich Nhat Hanh writes:

> Walking meditation is really to enjoy the walking—walking not in order to arrive, but just to walk. The purpose is to be in the present moment and, aware of our breathing and our walking, to enjoy each step. Therefore, we have to shake off all worries and anxieties, not thinking of the future, not thinking of the past, just enjoying the present moment. . . . If you feel happy, peaceful, and joyful while you are walking, you are practicing correctly.[3]

Swimming. The problem with swimming is swimming suits. The real difficulty there lies not so much in the suits or how we look in them, but how we think we ought to look in them. Self-acceptance may never have a tougher test than the swimsuit competition—the one in which the beautiful reality that you are today is challenged by advertising's persuasive image of how a body is supposed to look this year. Your growth in self-love will help you win in that internal swimsuit competition, and your new lifestyle will bring your body to its ideal state of health and fitness. Swimming—suit and all—can be part of that.

3. This quote comes from pp. 27–28 of *Peace Is Every Step* by Thich Nhat Hanh, listed in Appendix A. The author, a Vietnamese Zen master, offers detailed instructions there for walking meditation as well as for other helpful practices such as "Telephone Meditation," "Washing Dishes," and "Hugging Meditation."

When you swim, you feel light. Movements that would be labored if not impossible on land can be almost effortless. Swimming is an aerobic activity, yet it's also relaxing and conducive to contemplation. One winter I belonged to a health club equipped with an indoor/outdoor pool. I went in the mornings before work and felt incredibly accomplished when I showed up at the office knowing that I'd been swimming while snow fell all around me. If you plan to swim, be sure that the pool you choose has an atmosphere that's really pleasing to you. If the hours there aren't convenient, if the water is too cold (or, for that matter, if the staff is too cold!), you may want to look elsewhere.

Cycling. Bicycling appeals to my practical nature since it can be efficient transportation as well as aerobic exercise. If you can possibly use a bike for some of your commuting needs, I can almost guarantee that your life will change for the better in ways you might never have imagined. If you bike to work, your status in the company will improve even before your next promotion. That's because people are awed when someone actually demonstrates self-sufficiency, and getting to the job via person-power is self-sufficiency of the highest order. My fondest memory as a peddling commuter is whizzing past the bus I would otherwise have taken every morning. Of course, the same hill that enabled me to fly past a bus on my A.M. route, I had to huff and puff up in the evening. It was worth it.

Biking is excellent for the not-yet-in-shape because you can pace it to your fitness level from short trips on flat land to touring the Rockies. It helps to have a comfortable bicycle. The balloon-tire single-speed bike in the garage can provide you with a workout, but a bike with gears (a 3-, 5-, or 10-speed) can make two-wheel travel sheer delight. Being able to shift gears to compensate for hills makes for uniform energy expenditure as you ride. The result is less fatigue and more enthusiasm for the next outing. Don't think that a 10-speed means you have to ride leaning over. Those low handlebars are important for racers to cut down on wind resistance, but upright handlebars (available for any bike) are preferable for most of us.

Of course, who's to say how far you'll go? Some day you may want to race, or enter a triathalon, or get into mountain biking. Then again, you may prefer to pedal a stationary bike in your own family room while you watch a sit-com on the television. You get what you're after either way.

Aerobics classes. If you always wanted to be in the chorus line of a Busby Berkeley musical, you'll love aerobics classes. They provide the opportunity for anyone to dance, regardless of her number of left feet. (I say "her" because aerobics classes are overwhelmingly female, but men who summon the nerve to try it have a really good time. And, as you might imagine, the two or three men in a class of women are very popular.)

My preference is for *low-impact aerobics* which minimizes stress on the joints. Just because it's called low-impact, however, does not mean that a class is low-intensity. It can be quite intense and call for a well-developed state of fitness to be fun or, for that matter, effective. If a session is too difficult, it won't even be aerobic for you since you'll overexert and your heart rate will go beyond the aerobic training range.[4] Don't sign up for any classes you can't try out first. If a class is too tough and the instructor won't help you tone it down, find another.

Sometimes Y's and health clubs offer classes geared to beginners or senior citizens. I took a seniors' class when I was still in my thirties because it was the only one that fit my schedule. Along with weight training, that class put me at my highest ever level of fitness. I then made a cross-country move and haven't yet found aerobics as effective as that class. Why? For starters, it was easy enough to be fun. I enjoyed it, so I rarely missed a session. The teachers were friendly and down to earth. The participants encouraged each other. These are important qualities for you to look for in an aerobics program. Teachers should also be certified to teach aerobics and the facilities should accommodate this kind of class, with enough room for every student and a shock-absorbing floor to protect your knees and ankles as you exercise. Finally, music is an integral part of dance-aerobics. If you like the music, chances are you'll stick with the class—and you'll hum a lot the rest of the time.

---

4. Generally, aerobic training range is that place at which you're breathing hard enough to know you're exercising but not so hard that you can't comfortably carry on a conversation. For details about aerobic exercise, see *Fit or Fat?* by Covert Bailey, (Boston: Houghton Mifflin, 1989).

Weight training. Probably my favorite exercise, weight training is not usually aerobic[5] but the feeling of mastery that can come with every session is well worth having. Working with weights can also make profound changes in how your body looks in a very short time. Even more meaningful is how differently people start to regard themselves when they've been involved with weight training for a while. Instead of feeling weak or routinely taking the victim's role, a person who trains with weights notices a feeling of competence and confidence after only a few weeks. Strong people tend to feel strong, inside and out.

You can set up a home gym, but a well-equipped club can provide you with safety, instruction, and moral support. Working with a personal trainer who really cares about your progress can make up for all the unkind gym teachers you ever had. A short sentence like, "One more lift: I know you can do it!" can work wonders, not just for your deltoid or tricep muscles but for your sense of self.

Yoga. If you don't love your body yet, yoga can help you get to that point silently and surely. Hatha yoga, physical postures and breathing techniques, is thousands of years old. It comes from the Indian subcontinent but its benefits are not confined to a single country or belief system. Its slow movements, coupled with controlled breathing, result in a calming of the body and mind. Yoga develops flexibility of the entire body, particularly the spine, and it is believed to have various therapeutic applications.

Yoga was the first step I took in learning to love and care for myself. The technique I prefer for its gentleness and the consistency of its class routines is Integral Yoga. It was developed by Swami Satchidananda, an Indian teacher, and is taught at Integral Yoga centers and by trained instructors throughout the U.S.[6] This is the system employed in Dr. Dean Ornish's "Opening Your Heart" program in San Francisco. He writes this of yoga:

---

5. Heavy lifting requires rests between lifts and does not provide the steady breathing and heart rate elevation that characterize aerobics. Circuit training, using weight machines set at light levels, can be done continuously and aerobically. If you want to read something on weight training, I recommend *Getting Stronger: Weight Training for Men and Women* by Bill Pearl and Gary Moran, Ph.D. (Berkeley: Shelter Publications, 1988).

6. To contact an Integral Yoga teacher in your area, write Yogaville, Buckingham, VA 23921.

Actually, "exercises" may not be the best word, for these stretches are performed slowly and gently, with grace and control, as a type of meditation rather than as a form of calisthenics. . . . For most of us, the duality of our muscles—contracting and relaxing—is out of balance, for our muscles are chronically tensed and contracted. The first step toward experiencing inner peace and healing is to quiet down and relax the body.[7]

In my case, yoga also put me in touch with my body. I'd long tried to forget I had one because when I remembered that it was there I judged it as being fat or flabby or in some other way not measuring up. In yoga, I began to experience my body in a nonthreatening environment. The first thing I noticed was that I did have some natural flexibility. My self-image was then able to incorporate for the first time a positive trait that didn't have to do with being intelligent or having a good personality but one that belonged to my physical self. I also found my yoga teachers to be kind and patient. I remember one teacher saying, "Don't worry about changing your diet. Allow your spirituality to grow and *that* will change your diet."

If you're interested in yoga, visit a class and get a sense of it. Instructors of traditional hatha yoga (such as Integral Yoga) are adept at the slow, calming style of this ancient discipline. There are other styles of yoga that are rougher, even harsh. Some people do well with these, but if you don't feel better when you leave a yoga class than when you came, find another. Just as you'll need a soft mat to protect your back when you do yoga, your class should have an atmosphere that's like a cushion. After all, you're loving yourself to thinness, you may as well love yourself to fitness, too. When you approach your chosen physical activity or activities in this way, you guard against addictive exercise (see "The Exercise Obsession" at the end of this chapter) while you incorporate healthy movement into your life.

Love Yourself with Rest

Our society does not think too highly of rest and sleep. Resting is seen as laziness and sleep as a wasteful, albeit unavoidable, time expendi-

7. Dean Ornish, M.D., *Dr. Dean Ornish's Program for Reversing Heart Disease*, pp. 146–47. (See Appendix A.)

ture. We fit these in because we would collapse if we didn't but most people attempt to get around their need for rest and sleep any way possible.

Pushing ourselves—even with stimulants like caffeine—is accepted. Whether the goal is the honor roll or the executive suite, we give our work all we've got. That's fine up to a point, until we realize that "all we've got" is, physically, all we have! What we're talking about, this intangible substance that comprises "all we've got," is vital energy. The yogis call this life force *prana*. In martial arts, it's referred to as *chi*. Whatever we call it, it has to be regularly replenished. The natural way to do that is with adequate rest and sleep.

How much is adequate? It's enough for you to feel good. Most adults require about seven hours of sleep per night. You may need more, maybe less. One way to find out what's right for you is to stop using an alarm clock. Try this on the weekends first so you won't be afraid of being late for work and wake up at 3 A.M. wondering if you've overslept. After you've done this for a while, you'll discover that you have an exceedingly efficient internal clock. When you awaken to it, you'll be refreshed. Even confirmed night people become much more tolerant of mornings when the clock-radio is silenced and the internal clock takes over. (Don't worry about missing music in the morning: do this and you'll *sing*.)

If you have had trouble sleeping, many of the lifestyle changes recommended here may be helpful in that regard. People who have considered themselves chronic insomniacs have found that simply cutting out caffeine, not just in the evening but all the time, solves the problem. Exercise is also valuable. The body strives for balance (the fancy word for that physiological balance is homeostasis), so exercise naturally invites rest and sleep as its balancers. Meditation, too, produces the deep relaxation that encourages peaceful sleep.

Sleep isn't the only kind of rest we need. We are supposed to rest whenever the body gives us signals that it's tired. We've misinterpreted these signals in all sorts of ways. For most food addicts, tired feels like hungry. The message can also reach our brain sounding like, "It's time for a cup of coffee," "Work harder, lazy!" or "Everything is irritating me and I'm about to explode." The next time you get any of those messages in the midst of a busy day, take a minute to examine its content. Behind the hunger or the caffeine craving or the irritation might just be you, trying to ask yourself for a catnap, a little walk outdoors, a short conversation with another person, even a switch from filing to typing or vice versa.

When you have sizable chunks of rest time, be sure that your rest is really restful. Watching the news or a murder mystery on television isn't an athletic event, but it's not resting either. You can rest with a book, but you can rest more fully lying in a hammock watching the clouds. You can rest in a reclining chair listening to soothing music. You can rest by daydreaming, contemplating, unwinding in a bath scented with an essential oil like chamomile or juniper. Massage can also be sublimely restful. Honor your uniqueness by discovering those restful pursuits that make *you* say, "Ahh."

Love Yourself with Fresh Air

Take a deep breath. It feels good, doesn't it? Do it again and really blow out on the exhalation. It's a great feeling, relaxing and energizing at the same time. Our breath is our lifeline, although we seldom pay it any conscious attention. We don't have complete control over the quality of the air we breathe, but there are some actions we can take to breathe a little easier.

If you smoke, stop. Certainly this is a tall order because nicotine addiction is a powerful one. Whether you want to deal with your overeating or your smoking first, or whether you want to make both of those changes simultaneously is up to you. Smoking is generally regarded as a more rapid form of suicide than binge-eating, but to get all the life you're entitled to, get rid of both. Do not worry about eating more when you quit smoking! You are committed to loving and caring for yourself—your whole self. As long as you cling to any crutch to stay thin, especially a potentially fatal crutch like cigarettes, you won't know the freedom of *total* recovery.

Get the help you need to quit. According to Patrick Reynolds, director of the Foundation for a Smoke-Free America in Los Angeles, "Four out of five people who quit smoking today do it without being in a program, but later eighty percent go back. It's the same recidivism rate as heroin, so I believe it's important to participate in a stop-smoking program. The people who win in life are the ones who get help."

There are a variety of ways to get this assistance. The American Cancer Society and the American Lung Association both offer programs to help smokers become ex-smokers. Seventh Day Adventist churches and hospitals affiliated with them offer smoking cessation programs. (Their suggestions include cutting out red meat and caffeine to lessen the craving for nicotine, so Love-powered eaters are ahead of the game.) Smokers Anonymous, which uses the Twelve Steps, is growing. The most important thing is that you don't give up. "Most people have to quit several times before they stop for good," says Reynolds, grandson of tobacco magnate R. J. Reynolds and once a heavy smoker himself. "Don't lose your self-esteem, even if you've failed several times. The turning point for me was knowing I could not have even one cigarette, and in many cases it takes a program to impress that on people."[8]

If you don't smoke, stop smoking. In other words, don't breathe someone else's second-hand or sidestream smoke. It's hazardous to your health as well as uncomfortable. I've never been a smoker, but it used to be that when a hostess at a restaurant asked, "Smoking or non-smoking?" I'd say, "It doesn't matter." That translates as "I don't matter." But I do, and you matter just as much. You have rights. Stand up for them. This is especially true in your own home. If no one in your family smokes, it's my opinion that you don't need an ashtray. Your home may not be a castle, but it doesn't have to smell like a pool hall either.

Open windows, especially at night. We go so nonchalantly from central heat to central air that we forget there's another kind of air—the fresh kind! Letting some in will revive your spirits and having fresh air circulating in your bedroom at night can become a positive habit you'll never want to do without. Expect your quality of sleep to improve once you try this. (If it's winter, just open a window a little and use an extra blanket.)

8. The quotes from Patrick Reynolds come from a telephone interview with the author, April, 1991.

Give your household air a pollution check. Look in the yellow pages under "Environmental Consultants" or "Air Pollution Control" to find a company that can inform you about your indoor air quality. They'll check for pollutants such as radon (airborne particles of radium from decaying rock that are believed to cause lung cancer), formaldehyde (a suspected carcinogen that can come from carpets, paneling, and formaldehyde-foam insulation), and carbon monoxide as a combustion byproduct of fuels, as well as for dusts and molds that can aggravate allergies. If problems are found, there are ways (other than moving) to remedy them.

Don't be a domestic polluter. Improve your home's air quality by using environmentally sound household cleaners, commercial or homemade, to replace harsh chemicals.[9] Fumes from these (whether you can smell them much or not) end up in the air you breathe. (Just as using strong chemicals can decrease your air quality, having houseplants around can increase it by providing fresh oxygen.)

Do what you can to curb pollution in your community. Plant trees. Support clean air legislation. Become involved in local pollution control campaigns or back the people who are.

Treat yourself to "gourmet air" when you can. Gourmet air is the best there is—the sort you'll find in the mountains, in the woods, at the shore. Nature's most beautiful spots are also first-rate air purifiers.

Love Yourself with Water

You can love yourself with water externally and internally. We take baths and showers for granted, but have you noticed lately that it feels terrific to get clean? A shower is an invigorating experience, a bath is relaxing. Either one can be made special by using products that smell good and feel good. There's no reason why men as well as women can't treat themselves to scrumptious scents. The products that incorporate aromatherapy, oils that not only smell wonderful but are be-

---

9. For more on this, see *Clean & Green, the Complete Guide to Nontoxic and Environmentally Safe Housekeeping*, by Annie Berthold-Bond (Woodstock, NY: Ceres Press, 1990). Using strong chemicals in the home can not only pollute the air there, it can pollute the water elsewhere after it is disposed of down the drain.

lieved to have subtle, therapeutic effects on the mind and body, are not gender-exclusive.

Baths call for a lot more water than showers do. If you're going to take a bath, make it worth the water. Set aside enough time to really enjoy the process. Take the phone off the hook, or turn down the ringer if your answering machine is playing receptionist so you won't hear the call and turn your thoughts from your relaxing bath to "Who could that be?" (I've left a hot, fragrant tub to take a phone call that turned out to be a talking computer that wanted me to buy aluminum siding. Today, I'd give the bath priority.)

Do a little more with your bath than you think you deserve. It's good practice in stretching your ability to love yourself. Does it seem outrageous to you to light incense in the bathroom, or bathe by candlelight? Do it anyway! There's sick-outrageous—hiding chocolates under the water heater, forgetting that they'll melt—and there's well-outrageous—a bath with candles and music and a thick terry robe to slip into when you're finished. Food addicts are used to sick-outrageous, and in recovery we're eager to give that up. It's well-outrageous we need to get comfortable with. There's no better place to begin than in the privacy of the bath. (This is also a good place to start appreciating your body. Look at it kindly, touch it with care, and *talk to your body*. It will respond. See "Art Appreciation" at the end of this chapter.)

To love yourself internally with water, you'll need to obtain the purest drinking water you can. As hard as it is to believe, our bodies are more than half water, and the water we drink, like the food we eat, really does become *us*. You've no doubt read that it's good to drink lots and lots of water—eight glasses a day, even ten. We do need a great deal of water for our systems to function properly. If you're eating an abundance of fresh, raw fruits and vegetables, though, these are largely comprised of water, so you don't have to drink all the water you need. You'll be eating some of it. Generally, thirst is a fully efficient guide to when you should drink. The trick is answering that body signal with water instead of a soft drink or a beer.

Then there's the matter of what *kind* of water to drink. For most of us, tap water is not the best choice. Agricultural runoff and other pollutants enter the groundwater, which is then treated with chlorine in city water systems. Chlorine kills germs, but it does nothing to mitigate chemical pollutants. It is, in fact, a potent poison itself and it's only one of many chemicals that may be added to drinking water.

Intelligent options include purchasing bottled water (in glass containers if possible; plastic can leach into the water) or a home distillation unit. Distilled water is the purest kind. Dr. Joseph Weissman writes:

> What you *do* want is distilled water, and if that is not available, you may accept artesian or spring water. . . . Contrary to popular belief, distilled water *will not* leach minerals from your bones. Distilled water becomes thoroughly mixed with digestive juices as soon as you drink it. Once it is absorbed, it is no longer capable of acting differently from other body fluids.[10]

Use pure water for preparing all your foods and beverages, making ice cubes for everyday use, and drinking. If this water seems tasteless, that's because it is. Remember 8th grade science when we learned that water is colorless, odorless, and tasteless? Pure H_2O is just that, so some people don't like it. The alternative? Follow the example of prestigious restaurants by serving every glass of water with a wedge of lemon or lime. It's a gracious as well as a tasty habit. You can also try a splash of other fruit juice. An ounce or so is plenty. And when you're really thirsty—on a hot day or after exercise—straight, unadulterated water will be just fine.

We can also love ourselves with water by drinking it at the best times. Natural health teachers have traditionally warned against drinking with meals, claiming that water dilutes digestive juices and thereby impedes the digestion process. Some have also suggested that drinking with meals figuratively "pushes the food down," thus encouraging overeating. Their recommendation, then, is to drink half an hour before meals or two hours after.

I found that laughable. I never wanted to drink except at meals, but then I wanted to drink quite a bit. Being told "no" got to my rebellious streak, causing me too reach for the pitcher. Gentleness came through for me again, however, with the gentle suggestion I heard in a lecture by *Fit for Life* coauthor Harvey Diamond. He said that if you really

---

10. Joseph A. Weissman, M.D., *Choose to Live* (New York: Grove Press, 1988), pp. 55 and 62–63.

need to drink with meals, do it moderately, taking very small sips. That I could handle. I still drink with meals—probably more than is good for me—but I'm not a gulper anymore. And simple, summer meals made up primarily of fruits and salads are easy to enjoy with no beverage at all.

Love Yourself with Sunlight

Sunlight—enough, not too much—is a necessity for plants to grow, for children to grow, for life to exist on earth. We've been well warned about the dangers of excessive sun exposure. Particularly at this time in history when thinning of the ozone layer is causing more radiation from the sun to permeate the earth's atmosphere, baking your body in the sun is not just a cosmetic indiscretion; it could very likely lead to skin cancer. Nevertheless, you can also drown in water, exercise to the point of exhaustion, or rest so much that you accomplish nothing in life. This doesn't mean that you should never bathe, exercise, or rest. We need sunlight. We simply have to approach it with intelligence and respect.

A fascinating book on the subject is *Sunlight* by Zane R. Kime, M.D.[11] Dr. Kime cites scientific studies demonstrating the beneficial effects of exposure to sunlight in a variety of medical conditions. Unlike many of his colleagues who tell their patients to avoid the sun as much as possible, Kime recommends modest but regular sun exposure geared to individual skin type and the climate in which a person lives. One of his most fascinating contentions—one he documents from the scientific literature—is the sunlight/nutrition connection. He writes:

> Unless one has a proper diet, sunlight has an ill effect on the skin. This must be emphasized: sunbathing is dangerous for those who are on the standard high-fat American diet or do not get an abundance of vegetables, whole grains, and fresh fruits. Those on the standard high-fat diet should stay out of the sun and protect themselves from it; but at the

11. Zane R. Kime, M.D., M.S., *Sunlight* (Penryn, CA: World Health Publications, 1980).

same time they will suffer the consequences of both the high-fat diet and the deficiency of sunlight.[12]

Kime recommends a vegetarian diet of unrefined foods with ample representation from those rich in vitamins C and E and carotene, abundant in yellow and leafy green vegetables. A Love-powered eating plan meets these qualifications.

When you and the sun get together, use your head to give the best to your body. Here are some suggestions:

· Appreciate what sunny weather does for your disposition. When a day is really glorious, don't shut yourself off from it. Have breakfast on the patio, a walk during your coffee break. Take advantage of every beautiful day.

· For safety in the sun, remember Dr. Kime's dietary suggestions and stick with Love-powered foods, avoiding animal fats and most extracted oils.

· Remember "the golden mean" when you're in the golden sun. There is a difference between spending time outdoors on a bright morning or afternoon and lying on a beach at midday. One is safe and healthful, the other foolhardy.

· When you approach the sun, follow the "baby rule."[13] You wouldn't put a baby out in the noonday sun, but you wouldn't keep a baby indoors all the time either. Baby yourself.

Love Yourself with Emotional Poise

The body and the emotions are intimately connected and interdependent. Many of the physical practices we've alluded to in this section—enjoying the sunlight, getting enough rest, energizing with exercise—are natural antidepressants. Eating whole, natural foods also fosters emotional well-being because the brain is part of the body, nourished by the foods we eat. Sharp highs and lows in blood sugar levels precipitated by eating refined sweets can cause mood swings. William

12. From *Sunlight* by Zane R. Kime, M.D., p. 117
13. The "baby rule" comes from one of my healthy lifestyle mentors, Douglas Graham, D. C., of Club Hygiene, Marathon, FL.

Dufty refers to these as part of the *Sugar Blues*, defined in his book of that title as "multiple physical and mental miseries caused by human consumption of refined sucrose—commonly called sugar."[14]

Just as positive and negative physical actions can positively and negatively affect our emotions, emotions can in turn affect us physically. We've all experienced this body/mind interaction: feeling our faces flush when we're embarrassed, getting sweaty palms or butterflies in the stomach when we're nervous, salivating at the very thought of sucking a lemon or biting into a sour pickle. Most of us have also seen that bouts of compulsive eating can be tied to anger, fear, or some unidentified emotional malaise.

The science of *psychoneuroimmunology* deals with how the mind affects the body. It presents convincing evidence that love, joy, laughter, gratitude, and hope can prevent and may even help cure disease. The implication is that happiness doesn't just *feel* good. It *does* good.

No one could be happy all the time if that meant being elated, giddy, and ecstatic nonstop. No rational person would expect to sustain such an emotional peak. Besides, we couldn't if we wanted to: those extremes come in response to external events, events over which we have little (if any) control. The kind of happiness we can depend on is *contentment*. It's not exciting like elation, giddiness, and ecstasy, but it's only minimally dependent on outside happenings. We learned earlier that the body seeks to maintain homeostasis (balance). The mind does, too. When your mind is in a state of balance, contentment is commonplace. You can call it serenity, equanimity, emotional poise. By any name, it's great stuff.

Certainly, things can happen in life that could shake the serenity of a saint, but balanced people have a high contentment quotient and they quickly regain a comfortable calmness level. This occurs in spite of what is going on around them. Besides, it's not usually some major calamity that interferes with our contentment. "Nobody has ever tripped over Pike's Peak," my friend Mary Beth used to tell me. "It's the little stuff that will get you."

The starting place for dealing with this little stuff (and its bigger siblings) is the same place you started to deal with your food addic-

---

14. William Dufty, *Sugar Blues*. (See Appendix A.) The definition comes from the book's front matter.

tion: surrender, leaving the outcome up to God. Surrendering the outcome doesn't mean that we do nothing to help ourselves. An image shared with me recently was that of seeing our Higher Power as an orchestra conductor, ourselves as musicians. Musicians certainly don't "do nothing." They make beautiful music! But they do it under the direction of a conductor. Like those musicians, we're at our best when we do what we can and refrain from doing what we can't.

Two things we cannot do are change other people and avert natural law. Who would try anything that ridiculous? We would. We have! We've tried to change people by getting thinner (so he or she would be attracted to us), by working harder (so the boss would like us better), by being more self-sacrificing (so our children would appreciate us). We've attempted to get around natural law, too, usually the laws of physiology. "This box of cookies doesn't count because I'm starting a diet tomorrow" may sound familiar, as might praying to lose weight without giving up the food fix. When we stop trying to change others and circumvent the laws of nature, we can get busy with those actions that are ours to take on our own behalf. These actions bring us more emotional poise. They include:

Doing all we can to live in accordance with what we believe to be the will of our Higher Power. Peace Pilgrim, a remarkable woman who taught that inner peace was the prerequisite for world peace, was fond of saying, "Live up to the highest light you have, and more light will be given you."[15]

Allowing ourselves to be changed. Many of us have been self-help experts. We've done everything to change ourselves. Allowing ourselves to *be* changed is something else. The phrase that fits here is, "Let go and let God."

Performing the next task that is ours to do. The Buddhists have a lovely concept called *dharma.* It translates roughly as "duty." Every person has a dharma, a calling or purpose, distinctly his or her own.

15. Peace Pilgrim walked throughout the United States and in several other countries carrying her message of simplicity and peace from within. She lived the life of a spiritual pilgrim, having no possessions, walking until given shelter, fasting until given food. Since her death, her vision has been carried on by Friends of Peace Pilgrim, 43480 Cedar Ave., Hemet, CA 92344. *Peace Pilgrim, Her Life and Work in Her Own Words,* is listed in Appendix A.

We can work ourselves into a frenzy trying to do someone else's dharma, but when we're committed to finding and doing ours, a peace comes with it.

Treating ourselves with respect and expecting the same from others. We show self-respect with respectful thoughts about ourselves and respectful actions toward ourselves. Healthy self-respect does not allow us to play life roles such as the victim and the martyr. We learn to detach emotionally or separate physically from harmful relationships.

Learning to accept or change negative circumstances. Sometimes we need to temporarily accept a situation—a job that doesn't use our skills, an apartment with noisy neighbors—that can be changed later. We learn to do both these things by giving our highest good a priority.

In fact, changing and accepting are the only healthy options in any situation. We all know that deep down. That's why "The Serenity Prayer" (quoted in Chapter 4) has such universal appeal. C. Norman Shealy, M.D., Ph.D., a neurosurgeon turned psychologist who works holistically with patients suffering from chronic pain, degenerative disease, and emotional problems, says:

> I focus energy and attention on the things I can change and I choose to limit the number of things I try to change. Those things which can't be changed or which I've chosen not to change, I detach from and am serene, at peace. This is the ultimate goal: harmony with that concept. It's not to tolerate abuse or badness but not kill yourself trying to change what you can't. . . . If you choose to fight something, play it as a game. Enjoy it. If you choose not to fight, enjoy your serenity. Anything else creates problems. To be at peace, that's the goal. It isn't easy. It's just all there is.[16]

It isn't easy because we've grown accustomed to trying to control things. Even the phrase, "trying to control things," makes my jaw tighten and my shoulder muscles tense. Chronic controlling comes

---

16. This quote comes from a personal interview with Dr. Shealy in November, 1989, at his center, The Shealy Institute for Comprehensive Health Care, in Springfield, Missouri. The quote was first used in my article, "It's the Thought That Counts," which appeared in *EastWest* (now *Natural Health*) in March, 1990.

from taking what the authors of *The Answer to Addiction* call the "worm's eye view" instead of "the God's eye view."[17] A change in vantage point is needed for emotional poise to become typical for us. Most people cannot make the shift without help.

The Twelve Step programs are excellent resources for this help because the Steps are healing emotionally, as well as physically and spiritually. At least one organization, Emotions Anonymous,[18] uses the Steps for precisely this purpose. Practicing them to recover from a food addiction (or for any other reason) also brings about a noteworthy degree of emotional poise and inner peace.

In addition to a support group, professional counseling can be extremely useful. If you had counseling when you were involved in food addiction (whether you were practicing compulsive eating, or compulsive dieting), it may have seemed like a waste of money and time. Do consider it again if you feel the need. You're bound to find the experience far more meaningful when you enter it without the impermeable barrier of active addiction between you and the help being offered.

As you grow spiritually and live addiction-free, you are apt to find your overall stress level has decreased. Part of this will reflect a change in your attitude: there simply aren't as many things that drive you crazy anymore. And there will be fewer stress factors in your life simply because things will be in better order. (For example, you'll keep change in the car so you won't have to worry about having coins for parking meters.) If you need additional stress management techniques try:

· Meditation, affirmations, prayer

· Vigorous physical activity

· Massage and other bodywork

· Relaxation procedures such as yoga (the yoga breathing practices, in particular) and self-hypnosis

17. John Burns, et al., *The Answer to Addiction*. The phrase comes from the title of its 5th chapter, "The Worms-Eye View of Man—Spawning-Ground of Addiction." (See Appendix A.)
18. For information about Emotions Anonymous and meetings in your area, write P.O. Box 4245, St. Paul, MN 55104-0245.

- Play (see "Playtime!" at the end of this chapter) and laughter[19]
- Sitting with feelings
- Talking out feelings with another person
- Spending time in nature or with a companion animal
- Keeping a journal

These are wonderful practices, but I don't like the term "stress management." We've tended to manage everything far too much. I see gentle helpers like meditation and relaxation less as stress *managers* than stress *embracers*. The best information I was given for dealing with my daughter's fussiness during her "terrible two's" was to take her in my arms when she was out of control and hold her securely. It was sometimes a tricky maneuver—if you've known tearful two-year-olds, they can be pretty slippery—but it nearly always worked. Her sobs would melt into whimpers, her muscles relax, and we'd be able to rock and talk, pet the kitty, put the crisis behind us.

The techniques listed here can embrace stress in much the same way one can embrace a troubled child. When I do this for myself, whatever is causing me stress seems to soften, loosen, and let go. When I take the time to use any of the calming techniques available to me, I see I'm really embracing that childlike part of me. When that part in any of us is comforted and content, we really don't need much more.

◄ THE LOVE AND POWER OF COMPASSION ►

Compassion is a gift in the Love-powered life. If we were truly separate from one another, separate from the earth, and separate from our spiritual essence, selfishness would be the winning ticket. Compassion—that ability to "feel with" others—would be expendable. It could even be a detriment. As things really are, each of us only appears to be an independent entity. At a very basic level, we are a part of all human beings and a part of everything that exists. **It benefits us to think of others, not because there is some cosmic tally system of**

---

19. The best known work that explores laughter as a healing agent is Norman Cousins' landmark book, *Anatomy of an Illness as Perceived by the Patient: Reflections on Healing and Regeneration* (New York: W.W. Norton Co., In., 1979).

rewards and punishments, but because the compassion we share with each other is shared with the whole, ourselves included. For recovering food addicts, compassion is indispensable, because it is the opposite of selfishness. Addiction cannot exist without selfishness, just as fire cannot exist without oxygen.

Selfishness manifests itself in many ways. Surprisingly enough, self-effacement, self-denial, and self-hate are among them. These are not only negative and damaging, they're self-centered! Compassion, on the other hand, extends to those around us and to ourselves. It is all-inclusive. Our underlying connectedness makes this so.

In spite of the apparent separateness of everyone and everything, numerous individuals and entire civilizations have seen a fundamental unity within this diversity. The Native American world view has traditionally been one that has celebrated the interconnectedness of all life. The explanation of this given by Chief Seattle in 1854 has been quoted often, not only for its eloquence but for its truth that is timeless and cross-cultural. His testimony, given when his people were forced to give up their land, included this:

> We are part of the earth and it is part of us,
> The perfumed flowers are our sisters;
> the deer, the horse, the great eagle,
> these are our brothers. . . .
>
> This we know. The earth does not belong to man;
> man belongs to the earth.
> This we know. All things are connected like the blood
> which unites one family.
> All things are connected.
>
> Whatever befalls the earth befalls the sons of the earth.
> Man did not weave the web of life, he is merely a strand in it.
> Whatever he does to the web, he does to himself.[20]

Other people have come to an inner sense of this oneness in spite of, rather than because of, the society into which they were born. These people have had what we refer to as a spiritual experience, a unique state in which a person is intensely aware of the unity—and

20. Quote from *The Extended Circle, a Dictionary of Humane Thought*, Jon Wynne-Tyson, ed. (Fontwell, Sussex: Centaur Press, 1985), pp. 317–18.

some would say the divinity—of all life.[21] One of these was the late nineteenth century medical doctor Maurice Bucke, who wrote, "I saw that this universe is not composed of dead matter, but is, on the contrary, a living Presence . . . that . . . all things work together for the good of each and all; that the foundation principle of the world . . . is what we call love."[22]

Not only do those we think of as visionaries and idealists share this view; many scientists do as well. From the viewpoint of contemporary physics, Fritjof Capra, Ph.D., writes, "Quantum theory forces us to see the universe not as a collection of physical objects but rather as a complicated web of relations between the various parts of a unified whole."[23] And Albert Einstein is quoted as saying,

> A human being is part of the whole, called by us the "Universe", a part limited in time and space. He experiences himself, his thoughts and feelings, as something separate from the rest—a kind of optical delusion of his consciousness. This delusion is a kind of prison for us, restricting us to our personal desires and to affection for a few persons nearest to us. Our task must be to free ourselves from this prison by widening our circle of compassion to embrace all living creatures and the whole of nature in its beauty. Nobody is able to achieve this completely, but the striving for such achievement is in itself a part of the liberation and a foundation for inner security.[24]

All this isn't just entertainment for the intellect. No one recovering from food addiction can afford to waste energy on mind games. What comes from understanding our connectedness—perhaps intellectually at first, then at deeper and deeper levels of our being—is that

---

21. "Spiritual experience" is a broad term. I'm speaking in this paragraph of people who have had a particular, definable experience of heightened reality. If you are interested in these fascinating phenomena, I recommend *A Most Surprising Song*: The Mystic Vision by LouAnn Stahl (Unity Village, MO: Unity Books, 1992). Such an event is not required, however, for us to see life every day as a spiritual experience. I am reminded of the story of a Buddhist monk who said, "Walking on water is a miracle and walking on air is a miracle, but walking on earth is also a miracle."
22. Quoted in *Varieties of Religious Experience* by William James (Garden City, NY: Image Books, 1978), pp. 389–90.
23. Fritjof Capra, *The Tao of Physics, an Explanation of the Parallels Between Modern Physics and Eastern Mysticism* (Berkeley, CA: Shambala, 1975), p. 138.
24. Excerpted from an article which appeared in the *New York Post*, November 28, 1972, and quoted in the earlier cited book, *The Extended Circle, a Dictionary of Humane Thought*, Jon Wynne-Tyson, ed., p. 76.

our world view shifts from one of separatism to one of unity. When we see ourselves and everything around us as a unified body, we see ourselves and everything around us as important, valuable, and even sacred. With that vision, there is no forcing ourselves into compassionate behavior. We then *are* compassionate and cannot behave as if we weren't.

Compassion may be expressed in a variety of ways. When it becomes a factor in your food choices, as it is in a Love-powered diet, get ready for amazing things to happen. One of these was shared with me by Frances Moore Lappé, author of *Diet for a Small Planet*, the book that first suggested a reduction in meat consumption in the developed world to free more resources for feeding the hungry in all parts of the world. She said,

> Making healthy food choices for ourselves, other people, and the earth is empowering instead of punitive. I used to consider myself a compulsive eater. When I changed my diet—for reasons that had nothing to do with that—I started to learn about my relationship to food and the earth, other people, everything. Then I wasn't an overeater anymore. That was years ago. Since then my weight hasn't fluctuated more than two pounds.[25]

Choosing foods based on our relationship to the earth and our relationship to others reflects, in Lappé's words, "a larger vision. It's a shift from the idea of people as isolated egos battling for ourselves to a view of ourselves as beings in relationship." This larger vision makes compassionate living more than just a food issue. It touches every facet of our lives. Compassion is an *attitude* with *resultant actions*. You may take compassionate action in ways I haven't discovered yet. I may have come upon some areas of compassionate living that are new to you. We can learn from each other. Among the ways of incorporating more compassion into a life are the following:

Revise your definition of compassion. It isn't pity. It is not the province of the goody-goody or bleeding heart. The compassionate person has simply developed an aptitude for caring, like the artist develops an aptitude for painting. The only difference is that as human beings we *all* have an innate talent for compassion.

25. Telephone interview with author, July, 1990.

Enlarge your capacity to nurture. We nurture ourselves and others when we accept that all people and all creatures have needs, that it is all right to have needs, and that doing what we can to meet them can be fulfilling.

Retire as a judge. Stepping down from the bench relieves us of the responsibility of evaluating every person and situation in our lives.

Release your expectations. Addictive people often think they can save the world. We can't. We can do our part and release the rest.

Allow for the existence of pain. With enough compassionate people, the amount of pain in the world would be greatly reduced, but pain is part of life. John Robbins and Ann Mortifee write: "Our ability to feel compassion is greatly enhanced if we are able to be in the presence of pain—our own or another's—and yet still retain our balance and keep our heart open and calm."[26]

Permit other people to be themselves. Just because you change doesn't mean everyone else wants to. Resist the temptation to help them out too much. Perhaps their opportunity to grow hasn't happened yet.

Listen. Without giving advice, parading your wisdom, or trying to fix anything, listen to the other person. You can also listen to your body and to nature.

Extend your circle of compassion. "Until he extends the circle of his compassion to all living things," wrote Albert Schweitzer, "man will not himself find peace."[27]

Realize that little things count. One phone call can make a person's day. Recycling one aluminum can saves enough energy to run a television three hours.[28] Little things add up.

Become a compassionate consumer. We make purchases because a certain product is our regular brand, it catches our eye, or it's on sale

26. John Robbins and Ann Mortifee, *In Search of Balance: Discovering Harmony in a Changing World* (Tiburon, CA: H.J. Kramer, Inc., 1991), p.38.
27. *The Extended Circle: a Dictionary of Humane Thought*, p. 316.
28. *50 Simple Things You Can Do To Save the Earth*, p. 64. (See Appendix A.)

this week. Compassion can be as much an influence as habit, eye appeal, and price. Our buying habits have far-reaching effects. When we shop compassionately, we're also shopping *consciously*, freeing ourselves from the hypnotic lure of the marketplace.[29]

Treat yourself with compassion. When we ease up on ourselves, we tend to ease up on those around us. We expect less perfection from people and circumstances and appreciate the beauty in imperfect people and things.

Reflect from time to time on how your actions affect the whole. This doesn't only show you areas in which you might do better, it's also a reminder of the many areas in which you're doing very well. Seeing the beneficial impact your life is having can make you feel exceptionally good about who you are.

Make compassionate living an adventure. Being part of what a teacher of mine liked to call "the upward progression of the universe" makes life interesting, meaningful, and often lots of fun.

Trust that you'll be okay. The ability to show compassion is impeded by inordinate worrying about our own welfare. The antidote is faith. If "faith" sounds too much like Sunday morning, try Dr. C. Norman Shealy's definition: "believing that the purpose of life is good even if you can't figure it out."

Take the time to reach out. Everyone is busy, but our success doesn't necessarily correspond to how busy we are. Some of the most successful people are the least hurried. They know that there is time for what's important, and sharing compassion is important.

Give your compassion the opportunity to grow. Don't push yourself into actions that seem absurd to you. If, however, you find yourself catching an uninvited insect to release outside instead of reaching for the bug spray, don't think you've lost your mind. You may instead have found your heart.

---

29. If you're new to taking compassion to the shopping mall, you might appreciate the following books: *The Green Consumer: You Can Buy Products that Don't Cost the Earth*, by John Elkington, Julia Hailes, and Joel Makower (New York: Penguin Books, 1990), and *How to Make the World a Better Place: a Guide to Doing Good*, by Jeffrey Hollender (New York: William Morrow, 1990).

As we begin to see some of these actions being taken automatically and as we encourage ourselves to take other actions, it is crucial to remember that compassion is not a form of barter. It's not a way to get brownie points with God. **The fact that we're capable of living compassionately is itself a gift.** When my primary avocation was binge-eating, I was in awe of the people who seemed so effortlessly able to be available for others. They were literacy volunteers. They provided foster homes for stray dogs and cats. They planted flowers.

It was the ones who planted flowers that fascinated me most. They always seemed to be saying something like, "My begonias are out!" I never knew if they were on to something—I mean, is it really wonderful to have your begonias out?—or if they merely got a kick out of petty foolishness. It was when they brought cuttings around so everybody else could grow begonias that I got an inkling of what was going on. Planting something in the earth (compassion), watering and waiting (compassion), allowing a flower to bloom in its own time (compassion), appreciating its beauty and sharing that with others (compassion) is about as sublime a chain of events as this world can offer.

I wanted this in my life, but when I tried to emulate these people it never worked. It was like trying to stay on a diet. My version of compassionate living was to compulsively care for the rest of the world, ignore my own needs, and end up feeling resentful. Or I'd throw myself into causes and burn out before the first victory because I'd written so many letters, made so many phone calls, and attended so many committee meetings that I was too tired to care what happened. It became apparent that freedom from addiction, healthy balance, and the compassion that would make my life count for something would not result from my best efforts at self-improvement. Freedom, balance, and compassion were already within me, as they are in you. In the Love-powered life, they blossom—along with the begonias.

◀ THE EXERCISE OBSESSION ▶

Obsessive exercise is any fitness program that interferes with your life as a whole. New exercisers are often overzealous, but they soon become more moderate. Obsessive exercise, however, is not self-correcting. Like other addictions, it is progressive. Knowing whether you're exercising obsessively or just enthusiastically can be a tough call. One person who works out six times a week but can skip a day without regret if something important comes up is probably not obsessed with exercise. Another person exercising six days a week may rigidly stick to that schedule even when it means exacerbating an injury, rescheduling business appointments, and missing a son's or daughter's first softball game of the season. That's interfering with life.

If you're accustomed to exercising regularly, you feel a letdown without it. Your body and mind get used to steady doses of endorphins, the "feel good chemicals" that your system produces in response to vigorous activity. Your muscles become accustomed to exercise daily, or three times a week, or according to whatever other schedule you've set. And if you're doing exercise that you really like, you look forward to it as recreation as well. All these motivators are good because they make it easier to incorporate exercise into your life.

Obsessive exercise, however, is not motivated by wanting to feel good, having eager muscles, or enjoying recreation. It comes from believing that your worth is dependent upon how much you exercise. Many of us, particularly if we have been overweight or thought we have been, measure our worth with a scale, skinfold calipers, and a tape around the waist. The size, shape, and firmness of our bodies seem to be the most important indicators of our value as human beings. If we believe this, we no longer choose to exercise. We're forced to exercise. The exercise is healthy, but the motivation isn't. When we're pushed to exert ourselves beyond a reasonable point, the physical activity itself can also become detrimental.

Here are some questions to ask yourself if you think you might be an obsessive exerciser:

• Do I exercise when I'm injured?

- *Do I exercise when I'm sick?*

- *Do I exercise when it means skimping on sleep?*

- *Do I cancel social or professional plans to exercise?*

- *Do I skip meals to exercise (with or without compulsively eating later to compensate)?*

- *Do I feel guilty when I miss a workout?*

- *Do I keep close track of the results exercise is having on my body, by weighing and measuring myself persistently?*

- *Do I yo-yo from exercising a lot (seven to fifteen or more hours a week) to not at all?*

- *Do I ever purge or use laxatives to lose weight?*[30]

- *Do I exercise to make up for overeating?*

If you answered yes to two or more of these questions, you may be an exercise obsessive. If you answered the last question affirmatively, you could be exercising to rationalize binge-eating. This is particularly dangerous, because using exercise as an excuse to binge makes physical activity part of your food (and/or dieting) addiction. Juggling overeating (and/or undereating) with compulsive exercise is a trying performance. The inner changes that will arrest food addiction will do the same with exercise addiction. In addition:

Dedicate yourself to wellness, not thinness. *When overall wellness is your goal, a balanced life is more important than a rapid weight loss or flattening your abdomen in fourteen days.*

Guard against thinking of exercise in terms of calories utilized. *If you find yourself rationalizing extra food or a food you know to be harmful by telling yourself, "I'll take an extra aerobics class this week," you are on shaky ground. Use your spiritual principles and your support group to set your thinking straight.*

---

30. Purging (vomiting), laxative abuse, and compulsive exercise are bulimic behaviors, manipulative methods enabling a person to eat for a fix without the natural consequence of gaining weight. If you purge or abuse laxatives, you are a prime candidate for exercise obsession, too. Your recovery may well mean growing beyond these cover-up activities before your eating moderates on a consistent basis. Trust the process to deal with first things first.

Set a reasonable schedule for exercise and stay with that. *Three days a week should be the minimum, six the maximum. (Your body needs one day a week to rest anyhow, and having a day off can keep an obsession from developing.)*

Respect your body's current needs. *The body requires regular exercise, but circumstances can make other needs a priority. If you're in the acute stage of an illness, even if it's just a cold, you need rest, not exercise. If you're injured, you need to lay off a couple of days, or change the kind of exercise you do (switch from running to swimming, for example) until you've healed.*

Make exercise a part of your life as a whole. *Make some of your activity part of your family life (a Saturday morning bike ride, walking with your spouse, running with the dog) or your social activities (joining a folk dance club or a hiking group). Some exercise can also be incidental—walking to the grocery store or cycling to the office. When your exercise has more meaning than what it's doing for your hips, obsession is less apt to take over.*

Consider your commitment to exercise as a long-term one. *When you really believe that you'll stay active for life, it's not threatening to go easy or take a day off when you need to.*

Use some of your exercise time for nonexerting activities such as yoga, Tai Chi, or walking meditation. *Beyond the three weekly sessions of aerobic conditioning your heart deserves, you can choose from a variety of other aerobic and nonaerobic activities. If you're obsessive about exercise, you might rail against the milder pursuits that don't seem to burn enough calories to be worth the time they take. They will, however, slow you down so you can actually experience your body—an experience impaired by both compulsive eating and compulsive exercise.*

- - - - - - - - - - - - - - - -

◄ PLAYTIME! ►

Play is as essential for a healthy life as good nutrition, sleep, and exercise. It's an excellent de-stressor, can clear our thinking, and helps us put things into better perspective. Play and creativity are also inextricably linked. When we let our inner child come out to play, original thought often comes, too. "How do adults make themselves childlike without being childish?" asks Matthew Fox. "Play is the key. And art is the result of play."[31] You can lead a Love-powered life without play, but it won't be as productive—or as enjoyable.

A common complication of addiction is that it can cause people to lose their ability and even their desire, to play. Since food addiction can start in early childhood, some of us never fully expressed our inherently playful natures, even at that time in life when play comes most naturally. If we want to play now, we have to learn how to do it.

I was so serious about learning to play (in other words, about learning how not to be so serious) that I actually took a course in it: "Play for Grown-ups."[32] The teacher, a professional recreator, had us hanging from monkey bars and flirting with eternity from a jungle gym on the first night. Soon we'd worked our way up to hide-and-seek, Simon-says, and stacking ourselves into four-layer human pyramids at the park. It was terrifying! It was great.

In that class I learned that it isn't only overeaters who can have trouble with play. A lot of people are simply addicted to adulthood. With a strictly adult mind-set, play is extraneous, useless, nonproductive, a waste of time. It can even be a little scary. Science writer K. C. Cole stated in a New York Times article, "Play is out of control. In real play, we try things just to see what happens. In other words, we take risks." In adults-only thinking, risk is justified in business deals, the stock market, and if someone is drowning, but to risk making a fool of oneself with a Frisbee®—you must be kidding!

So don't start with a Frisbee. Start where you're almost comfortable. My teacher did warn against card games, board games, and sports at the beginning since they're taken way too seriously. Beyond

31. Matthew Fox, Original Blessing, p. 227. (See Appendix A.)
32. More and more adult education classes with this theme are being offered throughout the country at colleges, churches, and parks and recreation departments. I count the instructor of the class I took, recreator John Hutchinson, as one of the genuinely influential people in my life. Learning to be more childlike was a real growth experience for me, one that I recommend. I used the class as the basis for an article, "The Positive Power of Play," which appeared in the May 1990 issue of The Animals' Agenda. Some of the information here was first use in that article.

that, it's up to you. Here are some suggestions for gently reentering the world of play:

Develop a better opinion of goofing off. *A lot us have trouble with play because we really believe there's something wrong about not constantly working, worrying, eating, exercising, or being in some other way purposefully occupied.*

Rethink the idea of payoffs. *It's true that play does do good things for the mind and body, but it interferes with genuine playfulness if you're thinking, "This game of tag with my kid is reducing my work-related anxieties, developing a closer parent/child bond, and firming my quadriceps muscles."*

Come at play through the back door. *Befriend its cousin, laughter. Get some humor in your life every day. Read the comics. See a really funny movie. When you laugh, you're enjoying yourself without inhibitions. The same thing happens in play.*

Observe the play experts—children and animals. *After a while, you might even want to join in their games.*

Cultivate friends who are playful by nature. *They're the ones who seem to take life lightly. When you look for them, you'll find them.*

Liberate your own playfulness. *If you feel like singing when you walk, sing when you walk. They did it in Rogers and Hammerstein musicals all the time.*

Take a playful attitude into the rest of your life. *This isn't to say that there aren't times to be serious, but a person who knows how to play realizes that most things aren't nearly as serious as we make them. Because that person doesn't see every incident as infinitely grave, he or she can be most effective in those situations which really are.*

—※—

TEN

Forever

After

In a weight loss book, this would be the chapter on maintenance, on keeping it off. In a Love-powered life, however, these terms have little relevance. Maintenance implies continual, even laborious, upkeep, as in "The house was okay; it was the maintenance that killed us." And "keeping it off" is, if you think about it, a rather bizarre phrase. The implication is that fat reserves already burned for energy are somehow waiting to jump back on you like a friendly pup unless you're vigilant about "keeping it off."

Things can be different now. To start with, your job is not to maintain a weight loss. Only two percent of people who lose over twenty-five pounds keep from regaining the weight within seven years. Why go with odds like that? Instead, have as your job *maintaining your spiritual connection*. Then your Higher Power stays in charge and you stay addiction-free a day at a time. The old odds become meaningless, because your weight maintenance will be on a completely different basis.

Besides, now there is no weight loss diet to be followed by a maintenance diet. Love-powered eating is Love-powered eating. If you're normally a 130-pound woman and you eat what a 130-pound woman needs, you will eventually reach 130 pounds, whether you start at 135 or 150 or 300. You don't have to eat any differently when your weight reaches a certain point. There are also no formerly verboten foods to add back when your body is at a size that pleases you. The only foods you've chosen not to eat are those which are not loving to yourself and/or someone else. Being at a comfortable body weight isn't going to cause you to love yourself or others less.

But the most important reason that weight maintenance is not really an issue is that weight itself was never really the issue. It was an aftereffect. Love-powered living deals with causes. These are the facts:

- Addictive eating is an illness. It can recur. When conditions invite it, it will recur, regardless of body size.

- Like other addictions, this one has a spiritual solution. It involves surrender to a loving Higher Power, cleaning up our lives in general, and helping others.

- Living in this solution on a daily basis will prevent circumstances from developing that are conducive to relapse.

Living in the solution means continuing what works to help you live addiction-free. Practicing the last three of the Twelve Steps on an ongoing basis is an excellent way to ensure the spiritual growth that crowds out obsession. Those steps involve continued personal inventory, prayer and meditation, sharing with others, and incorporating spiritual principles into all aspects of living. It's wise to make these

Steps, examined in Chapter 4, a part of every day's activities—*even after you are thin*.

The tricky part about going on with recovery when your body is trim is that society has instilled in us the belief that food problems belong to fat people. In this instance, *ignore society*. It has not yet permeated the collective consciousness of humanity that food addiction is a disease of the spirit, which has *various* emotional and physical ramifications. "Many eating addictions are not visible," writes John Bradshaw in *Healing the Shame that Binds You*. "In the fat/thin disorder one obsesses on food constantly. The mental obsession is the mood alteration. It is really a mental distraction. By being in your mind and constantly thinking about eating or not eating, you can distract yourself from your feelings."[1]

Coming to grips with feelings through our spirituality and sharing with others can also be sidetracked if we're mirror-conscious. We can't take appearances too seriously. I once read about a movie star who said that he keeps his sanity (and his humility) by not putting much stock in his own press releases. Like him, we're better off not extrapolating from our success assumptions that aren't valid—for instance, that it is actually our success. We do take positive action and we can be proud of that, but we don't engineer our transformation. That's what our Higher Power does. A recovering overeater gave me her marble analogy for how this works:

When I was just beginning my recovery, I got an invisible marble bag with no marbles in it. After a while, I realized that the floor around me was covered with marbles—all sizes and colors. I started looking at them and realized that one was the cigarette marble. I picked it up, looked at it, and thought to myself that since I no longer chose to smoke I could put the marble in the bag. Then I saw the alcohol marble and since I don't choose to drink today, I put that in the bag. I put down sugar and placed that marble in the bag, then more foods as I put them down.

Then I looked around for character defects I'd been practicing all my life. By this time, I'd become aware of many of them and had let them

---

1. John Bradshaw, *Healing the Shame That Binds You*, p. 100. (See Appendix A.)

be removed, so I put the marbles for lying and gossip and some other things in the bag. It just goes on and on. When I'm doing what I need to do and letting God do for me what I can't do for myself, the string is drawn tight on that bag of marbles and I'm really enjoying life just as it is, not expecting, not anticipating, just enjoying.

Sometimes I stop doing some of the things that ensure good recovery—like reading literature that would help me, writing my feelings, going to meetings, sharing my secrets, talking with other people, and letting God be in charge of my life. Then some of the marbles start to roll out of the bag. At first I don't even realize it, but once I become aware, I can leave the marbles out to trip over, or I can choose to pick up and go back to what works. It isn't a bad thing that the marbles start to roll out: the trouble comes when I forget where they belong.

The ability to notice when we start to lose our marbles (so to speak) is the key to a lifelong reality of freedom from the food fix. If we could keep perfectly in tune with our Higher Power at all times, we wouldn't have to do anything else. But perfection among humans is rare at best, and trying to be perfect (instead of perfectly human) is a thankless task. We can, however, do our best to keep a strong connection with a loving God. When it's weakening, there are signs to watch for. Those that follow come from the insightful booklet, *A Look at Relapse*,[2] from the Hazelden Foundation:

- Exhaustion
- Dishonesty
- Impatience
- Argumentativeness
- Depression
- Frustration

- Complacency
- Expecting too much from others
- Letting up on disciplines
- Use of mood-altering chemicals
- Wanting too much[3]
- Forgetting gratitude

2. Charles W. Crewe, *A Look at Relapse* (Center City, MN: Hazelden Foundation, 1974), pp. 6–8.
3. Schooled in the tradition of hitching wagons to stars, I doubted that wanting too much was even possible. It came together for me when I realized that it isn't desiring that could get me in trouble—desires are good, they're our motivators—but the assumption that my desires are infallible indicators of what's best for me. In that spirit, there is a brief quote on my bulletin board from Rabbi Michal who lived in the 18th century: "My life was blessed because I never needed anything until I had it."

- Self-pity
- Cockiness

- "It can't happen to me"
- Omnipotence[4]

These signals apply to anyone recovering from addiction. Some signs I am aware of that are specific to food addicts are:

- Wanting to eat alone
- Eating larger quantities than usual at more and more meals
- Eating very quickly, taking big bites
- Biting nails; chewing hair, pencils, lots of gum
- Craving certain foods, or wanting some foods over and over
- Finding meals unsatisfying (the same meals that were fine last week)
- Control thoughts—"I'll skip breakfast," "I'll exercise more"
- New compulsions, i.e., overspending
- Return of old binge behaviors without the binge (yelling, lethargy, isolation, not keeping clean)
- Feeling suddenly that you have to lose more weight

Be aware that although these signs can be indicators of incipient relapse, they are not in themselves relapse. Seeing them is not terrible. It does not mean you have "blown" anything. In fact, seeing them can be good. These signals are like the abdominal pain that gets you to the hospital before your appendix bursts. They're the warning that something needs to change so you won't have to reenter the mire of guilt-ridden eating.

Like the woman with the invisible bag of marbles, we can go back to what works for us. It's smart to do that as soon as we realize that something is amiss. Food addiction is no game, and we cannot afford to play games with it. Even so, we don't have to be perfectionists and we don't have to be rigid. Among the joys of Love-powered living is that people *like* to do it. Being honest is liberating, prayer and medi-

---

4. In *A Look at Relapse*, each of these symptoms is explained in more detail. For this last one, omnipotence, the author writes: "This is a feeling that results from a combination of many of the above. You now have all the answers for yourself and others. No one can tell you anything. You ignore suggestions or advice from others. Relapse is probably imminent unless drastic change takes place."

tation are relaxing and comforting, and taking care of our physical bodies makes us feel good inside and out. **When the illness is rampant, none of this is motivation enough, but once recovery has begun, a sort of magnetic attraction toward wellness is established. You'll want to stay with what works.**

When you look at recovery as something that's for life, flexibility has to be there. Let's say that morning meditation is an important part of your Love-powered living. It's a weekday morning, you have to take the dog to the vet and the car to the shop, and you simply haven't scheduled enough time for meditation. Have you failed? Of course not! You can pray in the bus on the way to work and you can remember your Higher Power in all the activities of the day. This has been called "practicing the presence of God." You can be reminded of the wonder of life when you see a tree or a flower or a squirrel. You can feel the warmth of love when you're with your child, your mate, or a good friend. *And you can experience a miracle when you eat your lunch and it's enough.*

◀ FLEXIBLE FOOD ▶

Your food program has to be flexible, too. This is not license to eat for a fix, it's part of your protection from it. For medical, social, financial, or geographic reasons, you may have to make additional alterations at some point in the way you eat. For example, I hope that in my life I'll get to travel to China, to Africa, and to the South Seas—Java and Tahiti. Now I would imagine that the food is different in Java than it is here. As long as my spirituality is in good repair, I don't have to worry about food—in Java or my own kitchen or anywhere else.

Food addiction is serious and it can be frightening, but to worry about food (or anything else really) is counterproductive. For this day, God takes care of my food. To the degree that I allow Him (Her) to take care of the rest of my life, I have serenity. There is security in having a basic idea about what I'll eat today, but if that changes—if I end up eating at a restaurant instead of at home, for instance—it's all right. God can come to restaurants, too.

If a food situation is troubling, do what you need to. Pray. Call someone. Even leave. My experience has been, however, that when I gave up dieting for Love-powered eating, almost all food temptation went with it. I don't want to eat animals because I care about them. I don't want to eat animal food or junk food because I care about me. I want to eat and live in as loving and responsible a manner as I can because I care about the earth and about what is being left to my daughter and other children. Another recovering food addict who eats in Love-powered fashion explains it this way:

> I believe that God is extending His love and support to me, and that He wants me to spread it around to those I come in contact with—including animals. For me, this means not eating them. Also, I feel that the way I eat is healthful, and therefore nurturing. I'm able to be more nurturing to myself than ever, and how I eat is part of that. I want to be kind to myself, and kind to our planet and to God's other living creatures.

In this frame of mind, selecting some foods and bypassing others is no longer resisting temptation. With the help of a loving Higher Power, you get that desire-level healing that we talked about earlier in this book. When you have that, there is very little temptation to resist.

My life is better now than I could have imagined in the days of binges and remorse. That doesn't mean that it's perfect! For one thing, I'm a food addict. I'm not practicing the addiction, but it is essential that I pay attention to my spiritual life daily. Of course I need to do that to stay sane around food, but just as much I *want* to do it because it enriches my life in countless other ways—such as translating some of the general impulsiveness of my personality into creativity, energy, and enthusiasm.

My eating is not perfect either. It's best when I pay it very little mind: I eat, it's over, that's it. There are times, however, that I eat a meal, stand up, and realize I've had too much. There's nothing I can do about it except give the incident to God and forget it. Other times, I eat some food I know I don't need. I just want it. As long as I can eat it, enjoy it, and accept myself, I'm okay. If I started to develop guilt feelings, or if I wanted to continue eating, I'd need to get help—a prayer, a call, an honest talk with another person about ways I may have been deluding myself.

The same system works in other aspects of life. If something is making me uncomfortable, I need to look at it and talk about it. Food addiction does not mature in a vacuum, nor does it exist by itself. One of its functions is to protect us from feelings we couldn't handle. **Once the food addiction is out of the way, the feelings surface. This is normal. It's to be expected.** That's why many recovering people seek professional counseling. It doesn't mean that their recovery isn't working. It means that it is proceeding right on schedule. Until I understood this, I thought that having to deal with old issues negated the growth I'd made. Instead, I had to grow to be able to look at those issues.

◄ A SPIRITUAL WARRANTY ►

Something that all recovering food addicts (and anyone else who loses weight) has to look at is body image. How thin is thin enough? You can get some arbitrary weight from a chart or a memory ("I was 115 on prom night . . .") but I firmly believe that your body has the wisdom to settle at the weight necessary for its optimal functioning. If you exercise regularly, your body will also be less fat than it would be at the same weight were you sedentary. In any case, you will reach, and stay at, the size that is right for you by living according to the principles outlined in this book. *When you change your diet not with a specific goal weight in mind but because your life and your world will be better when you do, your body will take it from there.*

This may be the most difficult area of all in which to trust your Higher Power. I can remember hearing a talk by someone I greatly admired about trusting in the will of a loving God. I believed that God was loving and I'd long discarded the concept that tragedy and punishment were the ways that God's will manifested in my life. I just thought that God couldn't possibly understand about my body. I felt then that I had to be really slender and have those muscles that show—not big ones, just the kind that show because they're taut and aren't competing with fat for visual attention. I also had a goal weight that was as unchangeable as my date of birth or my Social Security number.

Well, I got to my goal weight. Then I went below my goal weight. Then I went well above it. Then I gave up the fight. My body found a weight at which it's comfortable. It's somewhat more than my old goal weight and a lot less than what I weighed when I insisted that the number I'd chosen on the scale was the only one I'd accept. I have no ironclad guarantee that I will never gain weight, but my body (and anything else that concerns me) is under a sort of spiritual warranty. The manufacturer takes care of it. The warranty is only invalid if I'm turning to food instead of turning to God.

Today's freedom, today's spirituality, today's contentment are all any of us gets. As we live in the way that makes these available to us, we have every right to trust that they will be with us forever after. The trust builds on itself. A recovering person says:

> The more I'm able to trust God and reach out to both God and other people for comfort and healing, the less need I have to eat when I am not hungry. I see my trust relationship with God (and with other people) as ongoing, something I will work at for the rest of my life. The paradox is this: I am afraid to trust—but the more I trust and put my life in God's hands, the smoother things go. Then it becomes easier to keep on trusting.

That's the trust that allows the power of Love into our lives, the Love that overcomes addiction and other assorted miseries. I have a sneaking suspicion, however, that just as we need to trust God, there may be ways in which God is trusting us. There are statues and stories, gardens and quilts, friendships and forgiveness that might never exist if we don't create them. There are people and animals and forests and rivers asking for our love and care. It could be that as we trust in a Higher Power to keep us free from obsession one day after another, that Higher Power is trusting in us to form the friendships and plant the gardens.

It's a collective effort, an effort that doesn't leave much time for agonizing over what to have for dinner or what you think of your thighs. Your dinner will be delicious, and your thighs will be just fine. The things you have to attend to are simply more important, more appealing, and more fulfilling. Not only will your meals be comprised of Love-powered foods, your days will be filled with Love-powered activities. With this combination, you will like living in your body, and you will love living your life.

❧ ART APPRECIATION ❧

The models in the fashion magazines have beautiful bodies. The guys on the team have beautiful bodies. The nudes in the paintings have beautiful bodies. You may feel singled out in having: no waist, flabby arms, sagging breasts, big hips, big thighs, big stomach, wrong proportions, and numerous other flaws. Mercilessly scrutinizing these, it's easy to forget that the models in the fashion magazines are often airbrushed adolescents. The guys on the team look no better than any twenty-year-old who works out. The nudes in the paintings do have big hips, big thighs, and big stomachs, but they're beautiful anyway because that's art. Excuse me, but you're art, too, and this course is art appreciation.

You've probably been told that a good exercise is to stand naked in front of a full-length mirror and experience the total impact of every lump, bump, and bulge. No. That's art criticism class. You've taken it every semester and you've passed with flying colors. Now you're enrolled in art appreciation. The concept is different. You're not supposed to judge the art (in this case, your body). You're supposed to understand it, find out what the artist had in mind in creating it, and learn why it is one of the greatest works of art of all time.

Your body is a great work of art because of its rarity, beauty, and value. We'll look at each of these.

Rarity. This comes from the fact that your body is one of a kind, unique to you. The unlikelihood of a certain sperm fertilizing a certain egg to result in your conception is, when you think about it, astounding. You are special—physically as well as in every other way.

When viewed in a universal sense, physical life itself is rare. Think of the vastness of space, the mind-boggling infinitude of an expanding universe. There may be life elsewhere, but as far as any of us knows for certain, this is it. That makes life on earth—your life on earth in your physical body—an extraordinary occurrence.

Beauty. The beauty of your body is a given. Nature is the most skilled artist there is, and every natural creation is beautiful. You claim your beauty the instant you decide to accept it as your birth-

right. I once interviewed a local actress who awed everyone. We saw her as talented, sophisticated, influential, and above all beautiful. I had been asking the typical questions when she leaned to within a foot of my face and said, "Look, I'm not really beautiful." I was shocked, but close up, I guess she wasn't really beautiful in the classic sense. She settled back in her chair and went on to explain, "Everyone thinks I'm beautiful because that's the impression I give. I figured out when I was very young that life would be better if I were beautiful, so I de-cided that's what I'd be. From then on I have been."

The last we heard of her, she'd moved to New York and married a producer, but it doesn't take a Cinderella story to make a person (man or woman) beautiful. We only think of ourselves as ugly when we compare the way we look to some arbitrary standard. For most of us, that standard comes from Hollywood or Madison Avenue. It's a stan-dard based on profitability, *not true human beauty. It's a standard with no roots in reality and one that is subject to change.*

Accept your beauty. It doesn't matter if you're overweight. At many times in history, plumpness has been considered attractive, and to this day in parts of the Middle East, full-blown obesity is a desirable at-tribute. I know, you don't live in the Renaissance or in the Middle East, it's healthier to be slim, and you want to wear nice clothes right off the rack. Of course. You deserve to be healthy and to wear what-ever you like, but that doesn't mean you can't love yourself today. As your life changes, so will your body. You may prefer to be thinner and that's fine, but you'll have no more ability to truly love your body when you're thin than you do right now.

Value. Whether you like your body or not, it is of great value to you, and to the people who love and depend on you. Appreciate it. Even talk to it. Say something like, "Body, you and I have been through a lot. I have a food addiction so you've been put through tough times along with me, but I'm surrendering that addiction now and putting it in the hands of a loving Power that can take care of me so I can take care of you. I've said disparaging things about you in the past, but I really do love and appreciate you. We're in this together."

You may feel strange talking to your body as if it were something separate from you, but food addicts are separated from their bodies anyway. Talking can help you come together as a healthy whole. The most important thing you can do to reach that end is to deepen your spiritual life every day. A recovering overeater and bulimic who has done this explains what has happened for her:

> I can really look in the mirror and like what I see. I attribute this to my daily meditation that listens and tells me I am not the sculptor of my form. The more I tune into my Highest Self instead of the ordinary, everyday, limited consciousness the more I realize who my Truest Self is. And I learn to love my body because that's what I walk in. I look at myself and the hurt child I was, and I thank my body for taking care of me so well.

Honor the rarity, the beauty, and the value of your body. You'll find that art appreciation can be a snap course.

- - - - - - - - - - - - - - - - - -

◄ FOR FOREVER AFTER ►

1. Never forget that food addiction is a disease. It can reactivate if you cease to nurture its spiritual solution.

2. Be honest in all areas of your life, especially about your food and your thoughts about food.

3. Stay with your support group, both for what it gives you and what you give it. There and elsewhere, cultivate positive, accepting people.

4. Keep up your spiritual practices, especially the last three of the Twelve Steps, which deal with continued personal inventory prayer and meditation, sharing recovery, and "practicing these principles in all our affairs."

5. Cherish your body. It is beautiful. If you can't accept your body as it is, get help from people who have accepted theirs.

6. Look out for the signs that your spiritual life may need your attention, and make the necessary changes.

7. Give your continued health as a whole person a high priority. This includes your physical health, your emotional well-being, your relationships, your work, your finances, and so forth.

8. Keep your eating flexible and livable. Avoid animal foods and

most high-fat foods; this will replace punitive diets with life-affirming, Love-powered eating.

9. Exercise regularly in ways that add to the overall quality of your life.

10. Express gratitude—to God, to life, and to people. Every addict in recovery is a visible miracle. It's easy to get involved with living and forget that. By all means be involved with living, but once a day, remember.

—❧❦—

APPENDIX A

Suggested

Reading

There are probably hundreds of excellent books from which to choose that deal with the various topics discussed here. Some of these books were mentioned or quoted in the text. Those that are not in the following list have their titles, authors, and publication data included throughout this book in the footnotes that refer to them. So, you can easily find information on those books that interest you.

This list, however, is a short one. Because I really hope that you read each of these, it would be ridiculous to recommend fifty books, although that many and more are certainly worthy of recommendation.

The ones I'm suggesting in this Appendix were chosen for four reasons: they provide information in keeping with that in *The Love-Powered Diet*; I believe they can be particularly useful for readers of *The Love-Powered Diet*; most are easy to find; and together they can comprise the basis of a Love-powered library. The inclusion of a book on this list does not imply that I endorse every concept in it. Each of these books, however, does contain information that has been helpful to me and that I trust can help you as well.

◄▓ BOOKS ON RECOVERY, SPIRITUALITY, SELF-HELP ▓►

Anonymous. *Alcoholics Anonymous*. New York: Alcoholics Anonymous World Service, 1976. This is the basic text of Alcoholics Anonymous and the foundation for all the Twelve Step programs.

Anonymous. *For Today*. Torrance, CA: Overeaters Anonymous, Inc., 1982. A lovely little volume of daily meditations specifically for overeaters.

Anonymous. *The Twelve Steps of Overeaters Anonymous*. Torrance, CA: Overeaters Anonymous, Inc., 1990. Details the Twelve Steps for overeaters.

Anonymous. *The Twelve Steps and Twelve Traditions*. New York: Alcoholics Anonymous World Service, 1953. A detailed exploration by one of the co-founders of AA.

Bradshaw, John. *Healing the Shame That Binds You*. Deerfield Beach, FL: Health Communications, 1988. Eye-opening look at shame as underlying issue in addiction and other life problems. Offers the Twelve Steps as solution plus helpful exercises and techniques.

Burns, John, and three other recovered alcoholics. *The Answer to Addiction: The Path to Recovery from Alcohol, Drug, Food & Sexual Dependencies*. New York: Crossroad Publishing Co., 1990. A profound explanation of addiction and its Answer using the Twelve Steps.

Dunn, Amy E. *Night Light, a Book of Nighttime Meditations*. Center City, MN: Hazelden, 1986. A little meditation for every night of the year.

Fox, Arnold, M.D., and Barry Fox, Ph.D. *Wake Up! You're Alive*. Deerfield Beach, Fl: Health Communications, Inc., 1988. A really happy handbook for positive thinking and bringing enthusiasm, belief, love, forgiveness, and perseverance into your life.

Fox, Matthew. *Original Blessing, a Primer in Creation Spirituality*. P.O. Drawer 2860, Santa Fe, NM: Bear & Company, 1984. Introduces the inspiring concept of Creation Spirituality, that divinity permeates all that is.

Nhat Hanh, Thich. *Peace Is Every Step, the Path of Mindfulness in Everyday Life*. New York: Bantam, 1991. A compassionate guide for bringing spirituality into practicality, for merging our spiritual lives and our everyday lives into one.

Pilgrim, Peace. *Peace Pilgrim, Her Life and Work in Her Own Words*. Santa Fe, NM: Ocean Tree Books, 1983. Peace Pilgrim was able to couch great truth in friendly conversation and engaging stories. This book does precisely that.

Roth, Geneen. *Feeding the Hungry Heart*. New York: NAL-Dutton, 1989. There's something on nearly every page to help you accept, appreciate, and trust yourself more.

◄ BOOKS ON NUTRITION, VEGETARIANISM, ► AND LIFESTYLE

Barnard, Neal D. *The Power of Your Plate*. Summertown, TN: The Book Publishing Co., 1990. Interviews with prominent medical doctors and scientists on food and nutrition.

Diamond, Harvey, and Marilyn Diamond. *Fit for Life*. New York: Warner Books, 1983. Introduction to the dietary principles of Natural Hygiene including excellent recipe section.

Diamond, Harvey, and Marilyn Diamond. *Fit for Life II: Living Health*. New York: Warner Books, 1987. Complete lifestyle guide covering all areas of natural, healthful living.

Dufty, William. *Sugar Blues*. New York: Warner Books, 1975. Exposé on sugar and guide for living without it.

The EarthWorks Group. *50 Simple Things You Can Do to Save the Earth*. Berkeley: EarthWorks Press, 1989. Handy guide to environmentally sound living.

Klaper, Michael, M.D. *Vegan Nutrition: Pure and Simple*. Paia, Maui: Gentle World, Inc., 1987. Nutritional guide to total vegetarianism.

McDougall, John, M.D., and Mary McDougall. *The McDougall Plan for Super Health and Life-Long Weight Loss.* Clinton, NJ: New Win Publishers, 1983. Well-documented examination of lowfat, starch-based, vegetarian diet.

McDougall, John, M.D., with recipes by Mary McDougall. *The McDougall Program: Twelve Days to Dynamic Health.* New York: New American Library, 1990. Takes readers through twelve-day health improvement program patients experience in the McDougall Program at St. Helena Hospital, Deer Park, CA.

Ornish, Dean, M.D. *Dr. Dean Ornish's Program for Reversing Heart Disease.* New York: Random House, 1990. Inviting guide to diet, exercise, and emotional well-being from the physician first to show that heart disease can be reversed.

Robbins, John. *Diet for a New America.* Walpole, NH: Stillpoint Publishing, 1987. Compelling volume exploring the positive impact of a totally vegetarian diet on other animals, our own health, and the health of the planet.

—✥✥✥—

Cookbooks

and

Selected Recipes

People think I'm a good cook, but really I'm just a good reader. With one or two superb vegan cookbooks in your possession and a willingness to try new things, you can start creating healthful, delicious, Love-powered meals *immediately*. Since you may not have access to a superb vegan cookbook at this moment, I've chosen sample recipes from a variety of them to get you started.

There are dozens, perhaps over a hundred, well-written, attractive vegetarian cookbooks on the market. I'm keeping my recommendations down to the ones I use in my own kitchen and can personally vouch for. These are completely vegetarian (no fish, eggs, or dairy), use whole rather than refined foods, have simple instructions, and call for readily available ingredients.

Cookbooks are not the only sources of Love-powered recipes, however. You can also find them in magazines such as *Vegetarian Times* (P.O. Box 570, Oak Park, IL 60603), *EastWest* (17 Station St., P.O. Box 1200, Brookline Village, MA 02147), and *Total Health* (Trio Publications, Suite 300, 6001 Topanga Canyon Blvd., Woodland Hills, CA 91367). New recipes also routinely make their debuts in the membership journals of the vegetarian organizations listed in Appendix C. *Guide to Healthy Eating* from Physicians Committee for Responsible Medicine (Appendix C) provides recipes already printed on 3×5 cards in every issue.

Additionally, several of the health and nutrition books listed in Appendix A include recipe sections, some of them extensive. For example, *Dr. Dean Ornish's Program for Reversing Heart Disease* by Dean Ornish, M.D., contains a plethora of lowfat recipes from top chefs. *The McDougall Plan* and *The McDougall Program* by John McDougall, M.D., include the lean and luscious recipes of Mary McDougall.

And the next best thing to private instruction is to see the preparation of beautiful natural foods via video. Marilyn Diamond's culinary expertise is showcased is an excellent video, *Delicious Vegetable Entrees from the Fit for Life Kitchen*. This video features such zero-cholesterol main courses as Shepherd's Pie, Vegetable Lasagna, and Mediterranean Rice Salad. Renowned chef Ron Pickarski, O.F.M., can make you a Love-powered gourmet with his videotape, *Friendly Foods*. Also, both the American Vegan Society and the North American Vegetarian Society offer inexpensive, basic cooking videos taped at their annual conferences.

If you cannot obtain these videos or books through your local bookshop or natural foods store, contact one of the following mail order distributors:

The American Vegan Society
501 Old Harding Highway, Malaga, NJ 08328

The North American Vegetarian Society
P. O. Box 72, Dolgeville, NY 13329

Vegetarian Times Bookshelf
P.O. Box 446, Mt. Morris, IL 61054

Important: If you are a food addict for whom all this talk of cookbooks and recipes seems to be approaching dangerous territory, slow down. Take it easy. For now you may need to stick with simple foods that require minimal preparation. That's fine. As your recovery progresses, however, you will almost assuredly find that owning at least one of the following cookbooks and experimenting with the dishes in it can play a positive role in your recovery and in your healthy life.

◀ RECOMMENDED COOKBOOKS ▶

The American Vegetarian Cookbook from the Fit for Life Kitchen, by Marilyn Diamond. New York: Warner Books, 1990, 422 pages. A veritable encyclopedia of vegetarian food selection and preparation plus over 500 elegant recipes. "Steddas"—healthful stand-ins for traditional dishes—are great.

The Cookbook for People Who Love Animals, by the people of Gentle World, Inc. P. O. Box U, Paia, Maui, HI 96779: Gentle World, Inc., 1990 (6th ed.), 192 pages. A user-friendly volume with stay-open binding, lots of quick sautées, and a substantial section of "Side Dishes and Beginner Recipes."

Ecological Cooking: Recipes to Save the Planet, by Joanne Stepaniak and Kathy Hecker. Summertown, TN: The Book Publishing Co., 1992. Meatless Sloppy Joes, dairy-free Escalloped Potatoes, even Carob Hermits with no oil or shortening are among the hundreds of "real food" recipes in this well-designed cookbook.

Friendly Foods, Gourmet Vegetarian Cuisine, by Brother Ron Pickarski, O.F.M, Berkeley, CA: Ten Speed Press, 1991, 278 pages. A world class gourmet chef, Brother Ron makes food not just "friendly" but of *cordon bleu* calibre—the perfect choice for those who see food as fine art.

The High Road to Health, a Vegetarian Cookbook, by Lindsay Wagner and Ariane Spade. New York: Prentice Hall Press, 1990, 288 pages. I've never had a goof using this clear, inviting cookbook by actress Wagner and her co-author. The chapter "Entrées for the Meat Lover" is super for new or would-be vegetarians.

The McDougall Plan Recipes, Volume One, by Mary McDougall. Hampton, NY: New Win Publ., Inc., 1985, 122 pages. An oil-free, total vegetarian cookbook with ultra lowfat recipes that are also ultra-yummy. *Volume Two* (158 pages, also from New Win) continues a tasty tradition.

The Peaceful Palate: Fine Vegetarian Cuisine, by Jennifer Raymond. 284 Margarita Ave., Palo Alto, CA 94306: Peninsula Vegetarians, 1991, 125 pages. Beautiful to look at and delicious to eat, meals prepared from this ringbound cookbook range from family fare to company's coming.

Simply Vegan: Quick Vegetarian Meals, by Debra Wasserman. Baltimore, MD: The Vegetarian Resource Group, 1991, 224 pages. Easy-to-find ingredients and minimal preparation time in 150 uninhibiting, good health/good taste recipes. Each one features a complete nutrient breakdown, including amount and percentage-per-calorie of fat. 67-page "Vegan Nutrition" section by Reid Mangels, Ph.D., R.D., is an excellent reference.

Ten Talents, by Frank J. Hurd, D.C., M.D., and Rosalie Hurd. Box 86-A, Rt. 1, Chisholm, MN 55719: Dr. and Mrs. Frank J. Hurd, 1968, rev. 1985, 370 pages. Home economist Rosalie Hurd and her physician husband make healthy hearty in this classic, ringbound volume in its 43rd printing. This is *home cooking*—hot soups, crusty breads, ribsticking loaves and burgers.

The Vegan Kitchen, by Freya Dinshah. Malaga, NJ: The American Vegan Society, 1987 (11th ed.), 64 pages. Salt-free, sugar-free vegan recipes, a compelling introduction to the ethical and physiological reasons supporting this dietary change, shopping hints and more make this ringbound volume a fine first vegan cookbook. (It was my first and I still use it.)

Vegetarian Cooking for a Better World, by Muriel Collura Golde. Dolgeville, NY: The North American Vegetarian Society, 1985, 30 pages. An ideal, inexpensive starter, this pocket-sized cookbook contains some 65 winning recipes from which to create full meals (soups, dips, entrées, etc.), plus a full dozen breakfast items.

◀ RECIPES ▶

Breakfast Fare

Banana Milk
The Cookbook for People Who Love Animals

Basic Pancakes
The High Road to Health

French Toast I & II with Fruit Sauce
The Vegan Kitchen

Oatmeal Waffles, Millet Waffles
Ten Talents

Oil-Free Granola
The McDougall Plan Recipes, Volume One

Smoothies
The McDougall Plan Recipes, Volume One

Salads & Dressings

Aztec Salad
The Peaceful Palate

Easy Pasta Salad
Simply Vegan

No Oil Dijon Dressing
Ecological Cooking

Tofu Eggless Salad
The Cookbook for People Who Love Animals

Vegie Salad Dressing
The McDougall Plan Recipes, Volume One

Soups, Sides, 'Ceteras

Corn & Potato Chowder
Ten Talents

Cream of Cauliflower Soup
The Cookbook for People Who Love Animals

Eggplant Caviar
Ecological Cooking

Garbanzo Cheese
The Vegan Kitchen

Oil-Free Herb Sauce
The American Vegetarian Cookbook from the Fit for Life Kitchen

Steamed Greens
The Cookbook for People Who Love Animals

Stuffed Baked Mushrooms
Ten Talents

White Dill Sauce
Ecological Cooking

Entrées

Asparagus Quiche
The American Vegetarian Cookbook from the Fit for Life Kitchen

Baked Beans
The Peaceful Palate

Barbara's Kale Cream Sauce Over Pasta
Simply Vegan

Basic Oatburgers
Vegetarian Cooking for a Better World

Corn Tamale Bake
Ten Talents

Neat Loaf
The Peaceful Palate

Spicy Potatoes, Cabbage & Peas Over Rice
Simply Vegan

Stuffed Pumpkin and Bread Stuffing
The McDougall Plan Recipes, Volume One

Sunburgers
The Vegan Kitchen

Vegetarian Chile con Carne
Ecological Cooking

Sweets

Banana Bread
The McDougall Plan Recipes, Volume One

Dutch Apple Custard
Friendly Foods

Gingerbread
The Peaceful Palate

Karen's Creamy Rice Pudding
Simply Vegan

Poached Apples with Almonds
Vegetarian Cooking for a Better World

Breakfast Fare

BANANA MILK

1 banana
½ frozen banana
½ to 1 cup water
1 teaspoon sorghum
  (optional)
1 teaspoon vanilla (optional)

Slice the bananas and place in a blender. Add ½ cup water, sorghum, and vanilla. Add additional water gradually to reach desired consistency (either thick or thin is good).

Drink as is, or pour over granola, other cereals, or fruit.

VARIATION
Add 1 teaspoon carob powder with the water, for chocolate banana milk.
Yields 2 cups

BASIC PANCAKES

1½ cups whole wheat pastry
  flour
¼ teaspoon salt
3 teaspoons baking powder
1 tablespoon cold-pressed
  vegetable oil
1¾ cups soy milk

The secret to fluffy eggless pancakes is in beating the liquid ingredients until frothy.

Combine the flour, salt, and baking powder and sift into a mixing bowl.

Combine the oil and soy milk and whip for about 1 minute. Pour into the flour mixture and mix until thoroughly combined. Don't worry about the lumps.

Preheat a lightly oiled griddle or large skillet. When a few drops of water sprinkled on the griddle bead up and roll off, the griddle is ready.

Pour ¼ cup of the batter at a time onto the griddle. Cook at medium-high heat until the pancakes begin to bubble, about 3 minutes, and the bottoms are lightly browned. If the pancakes bubble up before the bottoms have browned, raise the heat slightly. Turn with a spatula and cook until the second side is lightly browned. Serve at once with natural maple syrup or natural fruit syrup.
Yields 12 pancakes

FRENCH TOAST I

¾ cup water
½ cup raw cashews
2 dates
2 tablespoons frozen orange
    juice concentrate
7 slices bread

Blenderize first 4 ingredients. Dip bread into mixture. Place on slightly oiled cookie sheet and bake at 400° F until golden brown on underside (10–12 minutes). Turn, and brown on other side.

    Serve hot with fruit sauce.

FRUIT SAUCE

2 cups grape juice or other
    fruit juice
2 tablespoons arrowroot
    powder

Simmer until juice thickens. (It will set into a jelly when cool.)

FRENCH TOAST II

1 cup soaked garbanzos
1½ cups water
2 tablespoons oil
Flavoring: herbs, onion,
    celery, carrot, etc.
6 slices of bread

Blenderize first 4 ingredients. Dip bread into mixture. Place on lightly oiled baking sheet and bake at 400° F until golden brown on underside (10–12 minutes). Turn, and brown on other side.

    Serve hot with hot stewed tomatoes.

OATMEAL WAFFLES

7 cups oats, quick
7 cups milk (soy or nut)
⅓ cup oil
2 teaspoons salt

Simple and delicious.

    Mix in the order given with a spoon. Let stand overnight before baking (or until thick). Have waffle iron piping hot. Bake 5–6 minutes. We make our batter the night before and let it stand in the refrigerator overnight. In the morning the batter is thick (oats have soaked up all milk). Do not dilute. Spread with a spoon onto waffle iron.
Serves 8–10

MILLET WAFFLES

Follow recipe above. Replace 2 cups oats with 2 cups millet meal. Bake in waffle iron a little longer.

OIL-FREE GRANOLA

3 cups oatmeal
1 cup wheat flakes
1 cup rye flakes
1 cup bran
½ cup raisins
½ cup chopped dried
   apricots
½ cup chopped dates
1 cup chopped dried apples
½ cup chopped cashews
½ cup raw sunflower seeds
½ cup raw honey
½ cup hot water
1 tablespoon vanilla

Combine all dry ingredients, fruits, and nuts in a large bowl. In another bowl, mix the honey, hot water and vanilla. Add to dry ingredients and mix well. Spread a ½ inch layer on baking dishes and bake in a 250 degree oven for one hour, stirring occasionally. Remove from oven, let cool. Store in covered containers.

   Helpful hints: Nuts may be omitted, use more wheat or rye flakes. Other dried fruits may be substituted for ones suggested. Be sure to stir every 20 minutes or so to keep the granola from sticking or burning.

Servings: 10–12 cups
Preparation Time: 10 minutes; Cooking Time: 1 hour

SMOOTHIES

SMOOTHIE ONE
2 bananas
½ cup apple juice or water
½ cup frozen strawberries or
   other frozen fruit
   (raspberries, blueberries,
   peaches, etc.)

SMOOTHIE TWO
2 bananas (frozen)
½ cup water or apple juice
½ cup chopped fresh fruit
   (papaya, mango, peach,
   pear, etc.)

SMOOTHIE THREE
3–4 bananas
1 cup water
2 tablespoons carob powder
2 tablespoons honey

Blend in blender until smooth.

These suggestions may be varied by adding more water to make the smoothies thinner, or using more fruit to make them thicker.

To freeze bananas, peel, wrap in plastic wrap, and place in freezer.

Servings: 2–4

Preparation Time: 10 min.; Cooking Time: none

Salads & Dressings

AZTEC SALAD

1½ cups dry black beans
3½ cups water
2 cups frozen corn, thawed
2 large tomatoes, diced
1 large green bell pepper,
 diced
1 large red or yellow bell
 pepper, diced
½ teaspoon crushed red
 pepper OR pinch cayenne
1 red onion, chopped
¾ cup chopped fresh cilantro

DRESSING

2 tablespoons olive oil Juice
 of 1 lime or lemon
2 tablespoons vinegar
2 garlic cloves, minced
½–1 teaspoon salt
2 teaspoons cumin
1 teaspoon coriander

Wash beans, then combine with water and simmer until tender (2–3 hours). Drain and cool. (Note: Two 15-ounce cans precooked black beans may be substituted, thus skipping this step.)

In a large bowl, combine beans, corn, tomatoes, bell peppers, crushed red pepper, red onion, and fresh cilantro.

Whisk together dressing ingredients and pour over salad. Toss gently to mix.

You'll love the colors as well as the taste. This may be made in advance and keeps well for several days.

Serves 10

EASY PASTA SALAD

1 pound pasta, cooked and
 drained
8-ounce package frozen lima
 beans, cooked
3 carrots, peeled and finely
 chopped
1 teaspoon dill weed
½ teaspoon salt (optional)
4 tablespoons eggless
 mayonnaise

Mix all the ingredients together in a bowl. If time permits, chill before serving.

Serves 8

NO OIL DIJON DRESSING

¼ cup water
¼ cup red wine vinegar
2 tablespoons Dijon mustard
½ teaspoon oregano
1 clove garlic, pressed
Salt and freshly ground
   pepper, to taste

Combine all ingredients and mix thoroughly.
Makes ¾ cup

TOFU EGGLESS SALAD

2 12-ounce cakes tofu
2 tablespoons tamari
1 tablespoon oil
2 small onions, diced
2 celery stalks, diced
2 teaspoons sea salt
1 teaspoon turmeric
6 tablespoons nutritional
   yeast

In a medium-size bowl, mash the tofu; add
the remaining ingredients and mix well.
Refrigerate to keep cold.
   Delicious with salad or as a sandwich.
Serves 4

VEGIE SALAD DRESSING

⅛ cup lemon juice
1 teaspoon pure vegetable
   seasoning
1 bunch parsley
½ teaspoon marjoram
1 teaspoon basil
1 green pepper
5 tomatoes
1 carrot
1 cucumber (peeled)
3 green onions
1 clove garlic

Chop vegetables, process in blender until
smooth. Add lemon juice and spices. Add a
small amount of water, if necessary, to make
dressing the right consistency.
   Helpful Hints: Good over a lettuce salad.
Use your choice of lettuce, add sprouts,
broccoli, zucchini, etc. or other vegetables.
Servings: 1 quart
Preparation Time: 20 minutes; Cooking Time:
none

Soups, Sides, 'Ceteras

CORN AND POTATO CHOWDER

Simmer until tender:
1½ quarts water
2 cups cubed potato
¼ cup diced carrot
2 teaspoons onion powder
1½ teaspoons salt;
¼ teaspoon celery seed

When tender add:
2½ cups creamed or liquified
 fresh corn
1 tablespoon oil OR 1
 tablespoon nutbutter
 (peanut or cashew
 blended with corn)
½ teaspoon savory

Bring to boiling point. Serve with soup crackers or bread sticks. Garnish with fresh parsley or celery leaves finely minced.

CREAM OF CAULIFLOWER SOUP

2 cups cooked brown rice
5 cups vegetable stock
1 head cauliflower, chopped
2 stalks celery, chopped
2 tablespoons tahini
¼ cup tamari
½ teaspoon garlic powder
¼ teaspoon basil
⅛ teaspoon red pepper

In a blender, combine the cooked rice with the stock; blend at a high speed for 1 minute, until creamy. It will take a few blender loads to do it all. Each time use ⅓ the entire mixture. Add ½ of the cauliflower and blend at a high speed for 1 minute.

Pour mixture into a large soup pot. Place over medium heat; add the rest of the cauliflower and remaining ingredients. Cook for approximately 1 hour, until the cauliflower is tender.
Serves 5

EGGPLANT CAVIAR

1 medium eggplant
½ cup minced onion
2 small tomatoes, chopped
   fine
1 teaspoon salt
¼ teaspoon ground black
   pepper
Juice of 1 lemon
2 tablespoons olive oil

Prick eggplant all over with a fork and bake in a 400° F oven about 45 minutes, until very soft and slightly imploded. Scrape out pulp and chop finely. Stir in remaining ingredients and chill before serving. Spread on crackers or on thinly sliced dark rye bread.
Makes about 2 cups

GARBANZO CHEESE

1 cup soaked garbanzos
   (from ½ cup dry)
½ cup Brazil nuts
3 tablespoons nutritional
   yeast
1 small tomato
2 sticks celery
1 carrot
½ teaspoon onion flakes
1 fluid ounce lemon juice
¾ cup water
½ teaspoon kelp

Mix the Brazil nuts and water in the blender, then add rest of the ingredients and blenderize well.

   Place in a double boiler over boiling water. Cover. Cook, stirring occasionally, for 40 minutes.

   Pour into heat proof bowl or pan that has been rinsed with cold water. Chill a few hours in refrigerator. Unmold, slice and serve.
Yields about 1 pound

STUFFED BAKED MUSHROOMS

12 large mushrooms
1½ cups or more bread
   crumbs
Very small can tomato OR 2
   large peeled ripe tomatoes
¼ teaspoon garlic powder;
   salt to taste
3–4 tablespoons chopped
   parsley
Finely chopped walnuts
   (optional)

Wash and stem medium-sized mushrooms. Pack with stuffing of bread crumbs and chopped walnuts mixed with a little nut-butter and seasoned with tomato puree, parsley, garlic powder, and salt.

   Place in a baking dish. Thread on oil and sprinkle on salt. Bake in hot oven 425 –450° F till tender.

WHITE DILL SAUCE

2 tablespoons arrowroot
   powder
3 tablespoons water
2¼ cups soy milk
1 tablespoon dried dill weed
1 teaspoon lemon juice
1 teaspoon brown rice syrup
Pinch nutmeg
Pinch white pepper

In a small saucepan, stir together water and arrowroot until smooth. Stir in soy milk and dill weed. Cook, stirring constantly, over medium heat until thickened, using a wire whisk to avoid lumps. Add remaining ingredients. Cook for a few more minutes. Serve hot. This sauce is wonderful on broccoli, cabbage, brussel sprouts, and cauliflower.

Makes about 2½ cups

Entrées

ASPARAGUS QUICHE

WHOLE WHEAT CRUST
½ cup whole wheat flour
¾ cup whole wheat pastry
  flour
¼ cup soft tofu (optional)
6 tablespoons sunflower or
  safflower oil
¼ cup ice water
Dash of salt

FILLING
1 tablespoon olive oil
½ cup minced green onions
2 cups cut asparagus, roll-cut
  or sliced in ½-inch
  segments
½ cup water
1 pound firm tofu
½ cup minced fresh parsley
2 tablespoons brown rice
  vinegar
1 tablespoon light miso
1 tablespoon prepared
  mustard
½ teaspoon dried marjoram
½ teaspoon dried basil

Sift flours, then place in a food processor
with tofu. With motor running, add oil until
mixture is a mealy consistency. Add water, 1
tablespoon at a time, until dough begins to
form a ball. Turn out onto a lightly floured
board. Knead briefly, then form into a ball.
Roll out onto a floured board from center
outward in all directions until you have a 12-
inch round ½ inch thick. Place floured
rolling pin in center of dough and roll dough
up over rolling pin. Transfer to a pie plate.
Fold edges under to fit pie plate and flute
with fork or crimp with your fingers. (For
baked pie shell, bake 15 minutes in 350° F
oven.) Cover with a towel and set aside.

Heat oil with green onions in a large
skillet. Add asparagus and sauté briefly, then
add water and simmer over medium heat
until tender, approximately 5 minutes.
Reserve cooking liquid.

Preheat oven to 400° F. Combine tofu,
parsley, vinegar, miso, mustard, marjoram,
and basil in a food processor. Add ¼ cup
water from asparagus and puree until
creamy. Fold asparagus into tofu mixture.

Pour into crust and bake for 30 minutes.
Allow to set at room temperature for 30
minutes before serving.

VARIATION
For a crustless quiche, pour mixture into a
lightly oiled 9-inch pie plate or 1-quart dish
and bake as above.
Serves 6 to 8

BAKED BEANS

1 pound (2½ cups) navy
    beans
1 red onion, chopped
1 15-ounce can tomato sauce
½ cup molasses
2 teaspoons prepared
    mustard
2 tablespoons vinegar
½ teaspoon garlic powder
1–2 teaspoons salt

These beans are cooked in two stages. First the beans must be cooked until tender; then they are baked in an oven or a crock pot with the remaining ingredients. Either way, the longer they cook the more wonderful they become.

Wash beans, then soak overnight. Discard soaking water. Place beans in a kettle and cover with water to 1 inch above beans. Simmer until tender, 2–3 hours. When tender, add all remaining ingredients. Transfer to an oven-proof dish and bake at 350° F for 2–3 hours.

Crock pot method: After soaking beans, place in a crock pot with water to 1 inch above beans. Cook on "high" until beans are tender. Add all remaining ingredients, and continue cooking on "high" for 2–3 hours.
Makes 8 servings

BARBARA'S KALE CREAM SAUCE OVER PASTA

1 pound pasta, cooked and
    drained
¼ cup soy margarine
2 tablespoons whole wheat
    flour
1 cup soy milk
3 tablespoons nutritional
    yeast
½–1 teaspoon each basil,
    thyme, dill, garlic powder
Salt and pepper to taste
10-ounce box frozen kale

Heat all ingredients (except pasta) together in pan over medium heat, stirring often, until kale is done. Pour sauce over cooked pasta and serve.
Serves 5

BASIC OATBURGERS

4½ cups water
½ cup soy sauce
⅓ cup oil or ½ cup nuts,
   ground
1 large onion, diced
1 teaspoon garlic salt
¼ teaspoon Italian seasoning
¼ cup flaked brewer's yeast
4½ cups (old-fashioned)
   rolled oats

Bring to a boil all ingredients except rolled oats. Turn down heat and add the rolled oats. Do not stir. Cook about five minutes. Then set aside to cool. Form patties with oiled mason jar lid. Place on oiled cookie sheet. Bake at 350° F for about 45 minutes, turning every 15 minutes. Serve with ketchup or gravy.

Makes about 20–25 medium-sized burgers

CORN TAMALE BAKE

In a skillet sauté till tender:
1 large onion, chopped
1 green pepper, chopped
3 cloves garlic
Oil to tenderize

Add:
3 cups canned tomatoes
1 box frozen corn (2 cups)
¼ cup chopped olives
½ teaspoon cumin
¼ teaspoon cayenne or
   paprika
¾ cup corn meal
Salt to taste

Simmer in skillet covered for 1 hour. Stir occasionally and add a little water if it gets too thick (up to ¾ cup water). Put in baking dish to warm over.

NEAT LOAF

1 cup cooked brown rice
1 cup wheat germ
1 cup quick rolled oats OR
  oat bran
1 cup finely chopped walnuts
  OR sunflower seeds
1 cup chopped mushrooms
1 onion, finely chopped
½ medium bell pepper,
  finely chopped
1 medium carrot, shredded
  or finely chopped
½ teaspoon each thyme,
  marjoram, sage
2 tablespoons soy sauce
2 tablespoons prepared
  mustard
Ketchup

The look and taste of meatloaf without the meat or grease. It is great topped with ketchup, or wonderful chilled and sliced for sandwiches. The mixture can also be formed into patties and fried for burgers, or used to stuff vegetables like bell peppers.

The vegetables should be chopped as finely as possible; a food processor is an invaluable aid in this task!

Combine all ingredients and mix for 2 minutes with a large spoon. This will help to bind it together. Pack into a greased 5" × 9" loaf pan and bake in oven at 350° F for 60 minutes or until lightly browned. You may wish to top the loaf with ketchup after 40 minutes, then return it to the oven to bake the remaining time. Let stand for 10 minutes before serving.

Serves 8–10

SPICY POTATOES, CABBAGE, AND PEAS OVER RICE

2 cups rice
6 cups water
5 medium potatoes, peeled,
  and thinly sliced
½ green cabbage
10-ounce box of frozen peas
  (or equivalent fresh)
2 teaspoons curry powder
1 teaspoon turmeric
½ teaspoon ginger
½ teaspoon garlic powder
⅛ teaspoon cayenne pepper
Salt to taste (optional)

Cook rice in 4 cups water in a covered pot over medium-high heat until done.

In a separate frying pan, add sliced potatoes to 2 cups of water and heat over medium-high heat. Shred cabbage and add to potatoes. Add peas and spices to mixture. Continue heating in covered pan, stirring occasionally, until potatoes are tender. Serve over cooked rice.

Serves 4

STUFFED PUMPKIN

1 medium pumpkin or large
winter squash
1 recipe of bread stuffing
(following recipe)

Cut off the top of the pumpkin or squash and save for a cover (as if you were going to make a jack-o'-lantern). Clean out seeds and stringy portion. Place bread stuffing inside, cover with top of squash. Place in a large roasting pan with 1 inch of water covering the bottom of pan. Bake at 350° F for 1½ hours.

Helpful hints: This makes a good main dish for a festive meal. Serve with mashed potatoes, gravy, assorted steamed vegetables and bread or salad.

Preparation Time: 15 minutes; Cooking Time:
1½ hours
Needs prepared bread stuffing
Servings: 6–8

BREAD STUFFING

1 loaf whole wheat bread
2 cups water
2 onions, chopped
2–3 stalks celery, chopped
1 tablespoon dried parsley
2 teaspoons thyme
1 teaspoon marjoram
2 teaspoons sage
½ teaspoon rosemary
2 tablespoons low-sodium
tamari

Cube the bread, place on a baking sheet, and toast in a 300 degree oven for 15 minutes. Combine the remaining ingredients in a saucepan, bring to a boil and cook for 15 minutes. Put the toasted bread cubes into a large bowl, add the cooked liquid and toss well. Cover with a lid or plate for 15 minutes to absorb moisture.

Preparation Time: 60 minutes; Cooking Time:
1½ hours
Servings: 6–8

SUNBURGERS

1 cup sunflower seeds,
  ground
½ cup grated carrots
½ cup chopped celery
2 tablespoons chopped onion
1 tablespoon chopped parsley
⅛ teaspoon basil
1 teaspoon arrowroot flour
1 tablespoon oil
½ teaspoon kelp
1 tablespoon chopped green
  pepper
¼ cup tomato juice
2 tablespoons wheat germ

Combine all ingredients. Shape into burgers.
Bake on oiled baking dish at 350° F for 15
minutes on each side.

VEGETARIAN CHILI CON CARNE

2 tablespoons olive oil
½ cup chopped onion
2 tablespoons chopped green
  pepper
1 (16-ounce) can tomatoes,
  chopped, with juice
1 (16-ounce) can tomato
  puree
2 tablespoons chili powder
¼ teaspoon salt
1 cup sliced mushrooms
1 teaspoon Sucanat®
  (optional)
2 small cloves garlic, pressed
2 (16-ounce) cans kidney
  beans, undrained

In a large soup pot, sauté onion and green
pepper in olive oil until tender. Add
remaining ingredients. Simmer, covered, for
½ hour. Uncover and simmer for another ½
hour. Adjust seasonings and serve.
Serves 4

Sweets

BANANA BREAD

8 ripe bananas
2 tablespoons lemon juice
  (optional)
½ cup honey
2 tablespoons applesauce
⅓ cup water
4 cups whole wheat flour
2 tablespoons defatted soy
  flour
1 teaspoon baking power
1 teaspoon baking soda
1 teaspoon vanilla (optional)

OPTIONAL ADDITIONS:
1 cup raisins or chopped
  dates
1 cup chopped nuts

Mash bananas and mix with lemon juice, if desired. Add honey and applesauce, mixing together. Add ⅓ cup water. In a separate bowl, stir together the dry ingredients. Add to the banana mixture. Add vanilla and other optional ingredients, if desired. Dough will be very stiff. Put the dough into a nonstick loaf pan. Bake at 375 degrees for 35 to 45 minutes. To test for doneness, insert a toothpick into center of loaf; if it comes out clean, the bread is done.

Helpful hints: This makes one extra large loaf, or 2 medium loaves. This is quick and easy to make with an electric mixer. If you have a nonstick baking pan, it will not be necessary to oil the pan.

Preparation Time: 15 minutes; Cooking Time: 35–45 minutes
Servings: Makes 1 large loaf

DUTCH APPLE CUSTARD

24 ounces (1 large jar)
  unsweetened applesauce
2 tablespoons agar flakes
½ cup Dutch Honey (see
  below for recipe)
¼ teaspoon cinnamon
1 cup soy milk
1 teaspoon vanilla extract

Combine the applesauce with the agar flakes, Dutch Honey (see below), and cinnamon in a medium saucepan. Bring the mixture to a simmer over a medium heat and cook until the agar is dissolved (10–12 minutes). Add the soy milk and vanilla, stir until well blended, and cook for a few more minutes. Pour the mixture into a lightly oiled 4-cup mold. Refrigerate until set (2 hours). Unmold and serve.

DUTCH HONEY

1 cup brown rice syrup
1 cup soy milk
1 cup Sucanat®
½ teaspoon vanilla extract

Pioneers of the American West used Dutch Honey when genuine honey was scarce. The recipe presented here is a natural foods version of the original recipe.

This recipe yields about 1½ cups of syrup. Refrigerated, it will keep for about two months. It is an excellent glaze for breads, pies, and other baked goods. It is also a wonderful dessert sauce for fruit, custards, and "ice cream."

Combine all ingredients, except the vanilla, in a medium saucepan. Bring to a simmer and cook until it is reduced by one half (about 90 minutes). Stir in the vanilla. Cool.

GINGERBREAD

½ cup raisins
½ cup pitted dates, chopped
1¾ cups water
¾ cup turbinado sugar or
    other sweetener
½ teaspoon salt
2 teaspoons cinnamon
1 teaspoon ginger
¾ teaspoon nutmeg
¼ teaspoon cloves
2 cups whole wheat pastry
    flour
1 teaspoon baking soda
1 teaspoon baking powder

This gingerbread contains no animal ingredients and no added fat, yet it is moist and delicious. Try serving it with hot applesauce for a real treat.

Combine fruits, water, sugar, and seasonings in a large saucepan and bring to a boil. Continue boiling for 2 minutes. Then remove from heat and cool completely.

When fruit mixture is cool, mix in dry ingredients. Spread into a greased 9″ × 9″ pan and bake at 350° F for 30 minutes or until a toothpick inserted into the center comes out clean. Makes one 9″ × 9″ cake.

KAREN'S CREAMY RICE PUDDING

2 cups pre-cooked rice
1½ teaspoons cinnamon
1 tablespoon vanilla extract
1 cup raisins
½ cup slivered almonds
    (optional)
3–4 cups soy milk

Mix all the ingredients together in a pot. Simmer until the mixture begins to thicken (15–20 minutes), stirring occasionally.

Remove from stove and serve hot or cold.
Serves 8

POACHED APPLES WITH ALMONDS

⅓ cup sliced almonds
24 whole cloves
6 medium golden delicious
   apples, washed and cored
½ cup apple juice
1 cup tofu sweet sauce
   (recipe given below)

Insert 4 cloves around the top of each apple. In wide pan, place apples in juice. Cook, covered, over low heat until tender, about 8–12 minutes. To serve, place each apple in shallow dessert dish. Top each with a spoonful of tofu sweet sauce. Sprinkle with slivered almonds, raw or toasted. Serve warm or at room temperature.
Serves 6

TOFU SWEET SAUCE

1 cup tofu (8 ounces)
¼ cup maple syrup
½ cup apple juice
1 teaspoon almond extract

Blend until smooth and creamy.

—❈❈—

APPENDIX C

Some

Helpful

Organizations

There are numerous organizations and publications that can be helpful to you as you incorporate the Love-powered diet into your life. To
avoid overwhelming you with information, this listing is brief.
Through these groups and through your reading, you will be led to
other resources as well.

American Natural Hygiene Society, P.O. Box 30630, Drawer L,
Tampa, FL 33630; bimonthly magazine: *Health Science*. Dedicated to
the principle that "health care is self care," the American Natural Hygiene Society teaches the principles of natural, healthful living includ-

ing a diet rich in fresh, natural foods from the plant kingdom, exercise, fresh air, proper rest, emotional poise, etc. ANHS publishes an attractive magazine for members, *Health Science*, offers books and tapes for sale, sponsors educational seminars around the U.S. and an annual international natural living conference.

American Vegan Society, 501 Old Harding Highway, Malaga, NJ 08328; quarterly journal: *Ahimsa*. Established in 1960, the American Vegan Society is dedicated to disseminating the principles of veganism (total vegetarianism with an ethical basis) to bring about healthier people, a healthier planet, and a more humane world. The organization publishes a quarterly journal, offers books and audio-visual materials for sale by mail, provides assistance and information for vegans and those interested in veganism, and sponsors a biannual convention.

North American Vegetarian Society, P.O. Box 72, Dolgeville, NY 13329; quarterly journal: *Vegetarian Voice*. Educational organization providing support and information for vegetarians and those interested in vegetarianism. They publish an informative journal, offer a large number of books for sale by mail, sponsor local chapters throughout the country, and hold an annual conference, Summerfest.

Overeaters Anonymous, P.O. Box 92870, Los Angeles, CA 90009; monthly journal: *Lifeline*. OA uses the Twelve Step program to help people who want to stop eating compulsively. OA is not a diet club and does not endorse any particular plan of eating. It deals instead with underlying causes. There is no charge for membership, no weighing at meetings, and no one is too fat or too thin to be welcome. In addition to offering guidance on the Twelve Step way of life, OA provides invaluable peer support and reassurance that you are not alone and that you can recover. Meetings are held throughout the U.S. and abroad. OA also publishes relevant literature.

Physicians Committee for Responsible Medicine, P.O. Box 6322, Washington, DC 20015; bimonthly publication: *Guide to Healthy Eating*. Active in health and research policy, PCRM provides nutrition programs including publication of *Guide to Healthy Eating* (Virginia Messina, M.P.H., R.D., ed.) containing informative articles and low-fat, totally vegetarian recipes; the Gold Plan, an institutional nutrition program; and the distribution of free educational materials.

The Vegetarian Resource Group, P.O. Box 1463, Baltimore, MD

21203; bimonthly publication: *Vegetarian Journal*. This educational organization has a volunteer committee of physicians and registered dietitians who aid in the development of nutrition-related publications and act as consultants in answering members' questions. One or more of these professionals reviews all nutrition articles appearing in the 36-page bimonthly, *Vegetarian Journal*. The VRG also supports local groups, provides outreach to professional organizations, and sponsors an annual conference and other gatherings.

APPENDIX D

The Twelve Steps

To follow are the Twelve Steps as they come from their source, Alcoholics Anonymous. The word "alcohol" in Step 1 and the word "alcoholics" in Step 12 can be changed to make the Steps read appropriately for dealing with your food problem.

1. We admitted we were powerless over alcohol—that our lives had become unmanageable.

2. Came to believe that a Power greater than ourselves could restore us to sanity.

3. Made a decision to turn our will and our lives over to the care of God *as we understood Him.*

4. Made a searching and fearless moral inventory of ourselves.

5. Admitted to God, to ourselves, and to another human being the exact nature of our wrongs.

6. Were entirely ready to have God remove all these defects of character.

7. Humbly asked Him to remove our shortcomings.

8. Made a list of all persons we had harmed, and became willing to make amends to them all.

9. Made direct amends to such people wherever possible, except when to do so would injure them or others.

10. Continued to take personal inventory and when we were wrong promptly admitted it.

11. Sought through prayer and meditation to improve our conscious contact with God *as we understood Him,* praying only for knowledge of His will for us and the power to carry that out.

12. Having had a spiritual awakening as the result of these steps, we tried to carry this message to alcoholics, and to practice these principles in all our affairs.[1]

1. *Alcoholics Anonymous*, pp. 59–60. Reprinted with permission of Alcoholics Anonymous World Services, Inc.

Index

Note: The Introduction and Appendices are not indexed. Footnotes are indicated by locator followed by "n."

Beans. *See* Legumes
Binge-eating, 21, 24, 66, 155, 244
    foods, 14, 100, 116, 165, 166
Body, 26, 56–57, 255, 257–259
Body/mind interaction, 231–236
Book of Tofu, The (Shurtleff &
        Aoyagi), 199
Bradshaw, John, 250
Bucke, Maurice, 238
Buckwheat, 180, 202
Bulgur, 202
Bulimia, 11, 14, 24, 116n, 244n
Burkitt, Denis, 126, 134

Caffeine, 99, 122n, 142, 224
Calcium, 117, 138–139, 149–150
Calories, 122–125, 141–142
Campbell, Stu, 210
Campbell, T. Colin, 127, 134
Cancer, 123, 124, 129, 148, 183
Canned goods, 178
Cantaloupe, 158
Capra, Fritjof, 238
Carbohydrates, 146–147
Carob, 180
Carrot Butter, Mary McDougall's,
        205
Carrots, 163–164
Cashews, 181
Cauliflower, 163
Causes of overeating. *See* Inner
        malaise
Centering, 35–36, 57, 92, 116, 154
Change, 13, 19–20, 142, 233,
        254–255, 259
Character defects, 250–251
    see also Personal inventory
Charlotte's Web (White), 45
Cherries, 157–158
China, diet studies, 124–125, 126–
        127, 136–137

Choice
    examples, 80–81
    and food, 102
    Now, 88–89
    recovery, 79–93
Cholesterol, 105, 122–125, 148
Club Hygiene, 161
Cobalamin. *See* Vitamins, B$_{12}$
Cole, K.C., 246
Comfort zone, 46–49
    see also Point Zero
Commitment, 33, 172–173
Compassion, 214, 236–242
Connectedness, 62–64, 154–155,
        213, 236–242, 247
    see also Higher Power; Spiri-
        tual Connection
Contentment. *See* Emotional poise
Control, 234–235
Cookware, 137, 206–209
Corn, 163, 203
Counseling, 85n, 235, 255
Couscous, 202
Crash dieting, 116n
Cravings, 12, 37, 83, 99
Culinary Basics
    cookware, 137, 206–209
    ecology, 210–211
    fat replacements, 204–206
    food preparation, 175–176
    grains, 165–167, 188, 200–
        204
    grocery shopping, 176–179
    legumes, 143–144, 167–169,
        195–198
    natural foods glossary, 179–
        182
    organic foods, 182–185
    potatoes, 191–193
    salads, 185–187
    sandwiches, 193–195

⊰ ABOUT THE AUTHOR ⊱

Victoria Moran has written about health, natural living, and vegetarianism for twenty years for such publications as *Vegetarian Times*, *East-West Journal*, *American Health*, *Yoga Journal*, *Total Health*, and *E, The Environmental Magazine*. She is currently a contributing editor for *Vegetarian Times*. She has spoken and given workshops on the Love-powered diet and lifestyle throughout the U.S. She lives in Stamford, Connecticut with her daughter and three devoted cats.

For information about a Love-Powered Diet seminar
in your area, send a stamped, addressed envelope to:

Love-Powered Diet Seminars
P.O. Box 180
Riverside, VT 06878

Cover design: Kathleen Vande Kieft
Text design: Christine Taylor
Typography: Wilsted & Taylor
Index: AMC Indexing